LEADERSHIP BY EXAMPLE

Coordinating Government Roles in Improving Health Care Quality

D0668114

Committee on Enhancing Federal Healthcare Quality Programs
Janet M. Corrigan, Jill Eden, and Barbara M. Smith, *Editors*

INSTITUTE OF MEDICINE
OF THE NATIONAL ACADEMIES

THE NATIONAL ACADEMIES PRESS
Washington, D.C.
ww.nap.edu

THE NATIONAL ACADEMIES PRESS   500 Fifth Street, N.W   Washington, DC 20001

NOTICE: The project that is the subject of this report was approved by the Governing Board of the National Research Council, whose members are drawn from the councils of the National Academy of Sciences, the National Academy of Engineering, and the Institute of Medicine. The members of the committee responsible for the report were chosen for their special competences and with regard for appropriate balance.

Support for this project was provided by the Department of Health and Human Services, the Commonwealth Fund, and the California Healthcare Foundation. The views presented in this report are those of the Institute of Medicine Committee on Enhancing Federal Health Care Quality Programs, and are not necessarily those of the funding agencies.

Library of Congress Cataloging-in-Publication Data

Institute of Medicine (U.S.). Committee on Enhancing Federal Healthcare Quality Programs.
    Leadership by example : coordinating government roles in improving healthcare quality / Committee on Enhancing Federal Healthcare Quality Programs ; Janet M. Corrigan, Jill Eden, and Barbara M. Smith, Editors.
        p. ; cm.
Includes bibliographical references and index.
    ISBN 0-309-08618-3 (pbk.)
    1. Medical policy—United States. 2. National health services—United States.
    [DNLM: 1. Health Care Reform—United States. 2. Government Programs—United States. 3. Quality Assurance, Health Care—United States. WA 540 AA1 I455L 2003] I. Corrigan, Janet. II. Eden, Jill. III. Smith, Barbara M. IV. Title.
    RA395.A3I4935 2003
    362.1′0973—dc21

                            2003001324

ISBN 0-309-51693-5 (pdf)

Additional copies of this report are available from the National Academies Press, 500 Fifth Street, N.W., Lockbox 285, Washington, DC 20055; (800) 624-6242 or (202) 334-3313 (in the Washington metropolitan area); Internet, http://www.nap.edu.

For more information about the Institute of Medicine, visit the IOM home page at: www.iom.edu.

The serpent has been a symbol of long life, healing, and knowledge among almost all cultures and religions since the beginning of recorded history. The serpent adopted as a logotype by the Institute of Medicine is a relief carving from ancient Greece, now held by the Staatliche Museen in Berlin.

*"Knowing is not enough; we must apply.
Willing is not enough; we must do."*
—Goethe

INSTITUTE OF MEDICINE
OF THE NATIONAL ACADEMIES

Shaping the Future for Health

THE NATIONAL ACADEMIES
Advisers to the Nation on Science, Engineering, and Medicine

The **National Academy of Sciences** is a private, nonprofit, self-perpetuating society of distinguished scholars engaged in scientific and engineering research, dedicated to the furtherance of science and technology and to their use for the general welfare. Upon the authority of the charter granted to it by the Congress in 1863, the Academy has a mandate that requires it to advise the federal government on scientific and technical matters. Dr. Bruce M. Alberts is president of the National Academy of Sciences.

The **National Academy of Engineering** was established in 1964, under the charter of the National Academy of Sciences, as a parallel organization of outstanding engineers. It is autonomous in its administration and in the selection of its members, sharing with the National Academy of Sciences the responsibility for advising the federal government. The National Academy of Engineering also sponsors engineering programs aimed at meeting national needs, encourages education and research, and recognizes the superior achievements of engineers. Dr. Wm. A. Wulf is president of the National Academy of Engineering.

The **Institute of Medicine** was established in 1970 by the National Academy of Sciences to secure the services of eminent members of appropriate professions in the examination of policy matters pertaining to the health of the public. The Institute acts under the responsibility given to the National Academy of Sciences by its congressional charter to be an adviser to the federal government and, upon its own initiative, to identify issues of medical care, research, and education. Dr. Harvey V. Fineberg is president of the Institute of Medicine.

The **National Research Council** was organized by the National Academy of Sciences in 1916 to associate the broad community of science and technology with the Academy's purposes of furthering knowledge and advising the federal government. Functioning in accordance with general policies determined by the Academy, the Council has become the principal operating agency of both the National Academy of Sciences and the National Academy of Engineering in providing services to the government, the public, and the scientific and engineering communities. The Council is administered jointly by both Academies and the Institute of Medicine. Dr. Bruce M. Alberts and Dr. Wm. A. Wulf are chair and vice chair, respectively, of the National Research Council.

www.national-academies.org

COMMITTEE ON ENHANCING FEDERAL
HEALTH CARE QUALITY PROGRAMS

Gilbert S. Omenn *(Chair)*, Professor of Internal Medicine, Human Genetics, and Public Health, University of Michigan, Ann Arbor MI

George K. Anderson, Senior Partner, New World Healthcare Solutions, Inc., Vienna VA

Gerard F. Anderson, Professor and Director, Center for Hospital Finance & Management, Johns Hopkins University, Baltimore MD

Stuart Baker, Executive Vice President, VHA, Inc., Irving TX

E. Andrew Balas, Dean and Professor, School of Public Health, St. Louis University, St. Louis MO

Charles R. Buck, Jr., Health Care Consultant, Former Program Leader, Health Care Quality and Strategy Initiatives, General Electric Company, Weston CT

Bruce Bullen, Senior Vice President and Chief Operating Officer, Harvard Pilgrim Health Care, Wellesley MA

Colleen Conway-Welch, Dean and Professor, School of Nursing and Associate Director, VUMC Patient Care Services, Vanderbilt University, Nashville TN

Gordon H. DeFriese, Professor of Social Medicine, University of North Carolina at Chapel Hill, Chapel Hill NC

Sam Ho, Senior Vice President and Chief Medical Officer, PacifiCare Health Systems, Santa Ana CA

Sylvia Drew Ivie, Executive Director, T.H.E. Clinic, Los Angeles CA

Arthur Levin, Director, Center for Medical Consumers, New York NY

Jan Malcolm, Commissioner, Minnesota Department of Health, Minneapolis MN

Elizabeth A. McGlynn, Associate Director, RAND Health, Santa Monica CA

James M. Perrin, Professor of Pediatrics, Harvard Medical School and MassGeneral Hospital for Children, Boston MA

Helen Smits, Visiting Scholar, Robert F. Wagner School of Public Service and Visiting Scholar, the Institute for Medicare Practice, New York University, New York NY

Douglas L. Wood, Vice-Chair, Department of Medicine, Mayo Clinic, Rochester MN

Reviewers

The report was reviewed by individuals chosen for their diverse perspectives and technical expertise in accordance with procedures approved by the National Research Council's Report Review Committee. The purpose of this independent review is to provide candid and critical comments to assist the authors and the Institute of Medicine in making the published report as sound as possible and to ensure that the report meets institutional standards for objectivity, evidence, and responsiveness to the study charge. The review comments and draft manuscript remain confidential to protect the integrity of the deliberative process. The committee wishes to thank the following individuals for their review of this report:

John C. Beck, Emeritus Professor, School of Medicine, UCLA School of Medicine, Pacific Palisades CA
Maureen Booth, Muskie School of Public Service, Portland ME
Joseph Cassells, Health Care Consultant, Bethesda MD
J. Jarrett Clinton, DHHS Regional Health Administrator, Atlanta GA
John Colmers, Milbank Memorial Fund, New York NY
Kathryn J. Coltin, Director, Clinical Measurement Systems and External Affairs, Harvard Pilgrim Health Care, Brookline MA
William Cors, Senior Vice President, Somerset Medical Center, Somerville NJ
David Dantzker, Wheatley MedTech Partner LP, New York NY
Robert Galvin, Director of Corporate Health Care and Medical Programs, General Electric Company, Fairfield CT

Thomas Garthwaite, Director and Chief Medical Officer, Department of
    Health Services, County of Los Angeles, Los Angeles CA
Charles B. Inlander, President, People's Medical Society, Fogelsville PA
Jeff Kang, Cigna Health Care, Hartford CT
David Kibbe, Director of Health Information Technology, American
    Academy of Family Physicians, Chapel Hill NC
David Lansky, President, Foundation for Accountability, Portland OR
Chris Queram, The Alliance, Madison WI

Although the reviewers listed above have provided many constructive comments and suggestions, they were not asked to endorse the conclusions or recommendations nor did they see the final draft of the report
before its release. The review of this report was overseen by **Neal A.
Vanselow** (retired), Rio Verde, Arizona, and **Judith Lave,** University of
Pittsburgh, Pennsylvania. Appointed by the National Research Council
and Institute of Medicine, they were responsible for making certain that
an independent examination of this report was carried out in accordance
with institutional procedures and that all review comments were carefully considered. Responsibility for the final content of this report rests
entirely with the authoring committee and the institution.

Preface

The American health care sector is in need of improvement. In recent years, distinguished panels of experts, academic researchers, and hospital and health plan accreditors have called attention to serious safety and quality shortcomings in American health care. In 1998, the Institute of Medicine's (IOM) Roundtable on Quality published a statement entitled The Urgent Need to Improve Health Care Quality. A 1999 IOM report, *To Err Is Human: Building a Safer Health System*, focused national attention on patient safety problems as a common cause of preventable deaths. In the 2001 report Crossing the Quality Chasm: A New Health System for the 21st Century, the IOM called for fundamental reform of the health care sector.

Against this backdrop, Congress directed the Department of Health and Human Services to contract with the IOM to conduct a study of the federal government's health care quality enhancement processes in six major government programs—Medicare, Medicaid, the State Children's Health Insurance Program, the Department of Defense TRICARE and TRICARE for Life (DOD TRICARE), the Veterans Health Administration, and the Indian Health Service. The IOM established the Committee on Enhancing Federal Health Care Quality Programs to conduct this study. Committee members brought to the effort expertise in quality measurement and improvement, organization and financing of health care services and care delivery, patient care, and consumer advocacy, as well as experience in directing government quality oversight programs and in responding to quality oversight requirements from the perspective of a health care provider.

Throughout its work, the committee strove to view the programs under its charge from the perspective of patients. A patient-centered perspective places a premium on coordinated care over time, across care settings, and across multiple payers—especially important for those with chronic conditions. Such a focus requires government programs and health care providers to unify and standardize their quality improvement efforts.

In this study, the committee addressed two overarching questions. First, is the federal government adequately carrying out its quality-related responsibilities to the beneficiaries of these six major government programs? Second, what steps can be taken to make government's quality enhancement processes more responsive to the needs of beneficiaries?

The Committee's overall conclusion is that the federal government must assume a stronger leadership role to address quality concerns. By exercising its roles as purchaser, regulator, provider of health care services and sponsor of applied health services research, the federal government has the necessary influence to direct the attention and resources of the health care sector in pursuit of quality. There is no other stakeholder with such a combination of roles and influence.

In assuming a leadership role, the federal government will attract many partners. The desire to help patients is what drives so many of America's brightest citizens to enter the health professions, whether as doctors, nurses, pharmacists or administrators in the public or private sectors. The satisfaction of contributing to improvements in the health of one's community often motivates service on health care boards. Concerns that consumers, employers, and taxpayers receive the greatest value for dollars invested in health care will motivate the business community to support quality improvements. Finally, few issues are of greater concern to the American public than their health and their health care. We all have a stake in improving America's health care system.

Gilbert S. Omenn, M.D., Ph.D., *Chair*

Acknowledgments

The Committee on Enhancing Federal Health Care Quality Programs wishes to acknowledge the many people whose contributions made this report possible. Special thanks to Caroline Taplin (Office of the Assistant Secretary for Policy and Evaluation) who provided ongoing support and encouragement throughout the project. Numerous other experts in federal departments, federal agencies, and other organizations served as important sources of information, generously giving their time and sharing their knowledge to further the committee's efforts.

In the **Agency for Healthcare Research and Quality,** they include Charles Darby, Nancy E. Foster, Nancy Krauss, Gregg Meyers, and Thomas W. Reilly.

In the **Centers for Medicaid and Medicare Services,** they include Rachel Block, Regina Buchanan, Eileen Davidson, Paul Elstein, Barbara Fleming, Lisa Hines, Tom Hoyer, Stephen F. Jencks, Jeffrey Kang, Steve Klauser, Patricia MacTaggart, Regina McPhillips, Dorothea Musgrave, Barbara Paul, Thomas Scully, Armen Thoumaian, and Sidney Trieger.

In the **Department of Defense,** they include D. E. Casey Jones, Marie-Jocelyne Charles, Daniel L. Cohen, Victor Eilenfield, Marion Gosnell, Bart Harmon, Bonnie Jennings, Pamela Jordan, Brian Kelly, Ben Long, Dan Magee, Reta Michak, Mark Paris, Jessica Powers, Geoffrey W. Rake, Jr., David Ray, Kimberly Roe, Teresa Sommese, Wyatt Smith, Frances Stewart, and Robert Wah.

In the **Health Resources and Services Administration,** they include Laura McNally and William Robinson.

In the **National Institutes of Health,** they include Nancy Miller and Molla Donaldson.

In the **Indian Health Services,** they include Angela Kihega, Edna Paisano, Robert Pittman, and Rosetta Tracy.

In the **Veterans Health Administration,** they include James Bagian, Darryl Campbell, Gary Christopherson, John Demakis, Noel Eldridge, David Gaba, Frances Murphy, Jonathan B. Perlin, Marta Render, Louise Van Diepen, and William Weeks.

Numerous other individuals made important contributions to the committee's work. They include Richard J. Bringewatt of the National Chronic Care Consortium, Suzanne Delbanco of the Leapfrog Group, Robert Galvin of the General Electric Company, Sheldon Greenfield of the New England Medical Center, Kenneth W. Kizer of the National Quality Forum, Kathleen Lohr of the Research Triangle Institute, Margaret E. O'Kane of the National Committee on Quality Assurance, Elaine Power of the National Quality Forum, James Reinertsen of the Reinertsen Group, Burtt Richardson of the Healthy Futures Partnership in Maine, Trish Riley of the National Academy for State Health Policy, Sara Rosenbaum of the George Washington University Center for Health Services Research and Policy, Thomas C. Royer of CHRISTUS Health, Matthew Salo of the National Governors Association, David G. Schulke of the American Health Quality Association, Shoshanna Sofaer of Baruch College, William Stead of Vanderbilt University, Edward Wagner of the Group Health Cooperative of Puget Sound, Edward Westrick of Rhode Island Quality Partners, Helen Wu of the National Quality Forum, and Ann Page and Elaine Swift of the Institute of Medicine.

October 2002

Glossary

Chronic conditions. A condition that requires ongoing medical care including monitoring, treatment, and coordination among multiple providers, limits what one can do, and is likely to last longer than one year. Examples include diabetes, cancer, and cardiovascular disease (Partnerships for Solutions, 2002).

Clinicians. Individual health care providers, such as physicians, nurse practitioners, nurses, physician assistants, and others.

Dual eligible. Individuals enrolled in more than one government health care program. For example, individuals who are beneficiaries of both the Medicare and Medicaid programs, or those receiving benefits under both the Veterans Health Administration and Medicare.

Government health care programs. The six government-sponsored insurance and/or health care delivery programs reviewed in this report: Medicare, Medicaid, the State Children's Health Insurance Program, the Department of Defense's TRICARE and TRICARE for Life Programs, the Veterans Health Administration program, and the Indian Health Service program.

Providers. Refers to both institutional providers of health care services (e.g., health plans, health maintenance organizations (HMOs), hospitals, nursing homes) and clinicians (e.g., physicians, nurse practitioners, nurses, physician assistants).

Quality. The degree to which health services for individuals and populations increase the likelihood of desired health outcomes and are consistent with current professional knowledge (Institute of Medicine, 1990).

Quality aims. Six dimensions of quality that constitute the goals of the health system (Institute of Medicine, 2001). They are:

Safe—avoiding injuries to patients from the care that is intended to help them.

Effective—providing services based on scientific knowledge to all who could benefit and refraining from providing services to those not likely to benefit (avoiding underuse and overuse, respectively).

Patient-centered—providing care that is respectful of and responsive to individual patient preferences, needs, and values and ensuring that patient values guide all clinical decisions.

Timely—reducing waits and sometimes harmful delays for both those who receive and those who give care.

Efficient—avoiding waste, including waste of equipment, supplies, ideas, and energy.

Equitable—providing care that does not vary in quality because of personal characteristics such as gender, ethnicity, geographic location, and socioeconomic status.

Quality enhancement processes. The range of activities—including review, certification, performance measurement, and technical assistance—pursued by government health care programs to assess and improve the quality of health care outcomes, structures, and processes.

Quality management activity (internal). The ongoing, organized activities of a provider that focus on measuring, monitoring, or improving the quality of services it provides.

Quality (or performance) measures. These include measures of patient perspectives on care, clinical quality, and patient outcomes.

• Measures of patient perspectives include patient assessment and satisfaction with their access to and interactions with the care delivery system (e.g., waiting times, information received from providers, choice of providers).

• Measures of clinical quality are specific quantitative indicators to identify whether the care provided conforms to established treatment goals and care processes for specific clinical presentations. Clinical quality measures generally consist of a descriptive statement or indicator (e.g., the rate of beta blocker usage after heart attack, the 30-day mortality rate following coronary artery bypass graft surgery), a list of data elements that are necessary to construct and/or report the measure, detailed specifications that direct how the data elements are to be collected (including the source of data), the population on whom the measure is constructed, the timing of data collection and reporting, the analytic models used to construct the measure, and the format in which the results will be presented. Measures may also include thresholds, standards, or other benchmarks of performance (McGlynn, 2002).

- Measures of patient outcomes include mortality, morbidity, and physical and mental functioning.

Quality review (external). Ongoing, organized reviews, conducted by independent external entities, of the quality of services offered by a health care provider. For example, states are required to contract with independent external review organizations to conduct annual assessments of the quality of services provided to Medicaid beneficiaries in HMOs.

Risk adjustment. A process that modifies the analysis of performance measurement results by those characteristics of the patient population that affect results, are out of the control of providers, and are likely to be common and not randomly distributed.

Safety-net providers. Providers that historically have had large Medicaid and indigent care caseloads relative to other providers and are willing to offer services regardless of the patient's ability to pay (AcademyHealth, 2002).

Vulnerable populations. Persons who are at increased risk of poor health outcomes. For example, persons with severe and chronic mental illness, the frail elderly, racial minorities, and the poor.

REFERENCE LIST

AcademyHealth. 2002. "Academy Publications: Glossary of Terms Commonly Used in Health Care." Online. Available at http://www.academyhealth.org/publications/glossary.pdf [accessed July 3, 2002].

Institute of Medicine. 1990. *Medicare: A Strategy for Quality Assurance.* Washington DC: National Academy Press.

———. 2001. *Crossing the Quality Chasm: A New Health System for the 21st Century.* Washington DC: National Academy Press.

McGlynn, E. A. (RAND Health). July 2002. Quality Measures. Personal communication to Janet Corrigan.

Partnerships for Solutions. 2002. *Better Lives for People with Chronic Conditions. Medicare: Cost and prevalence of chronic conditions.* Baltimore MD: Johns Hopkins University.

Contents

Tables, Figures, and Boxes

TABLES

FIGURES

BOXES

LEADERSHIP BY EXAMPLE

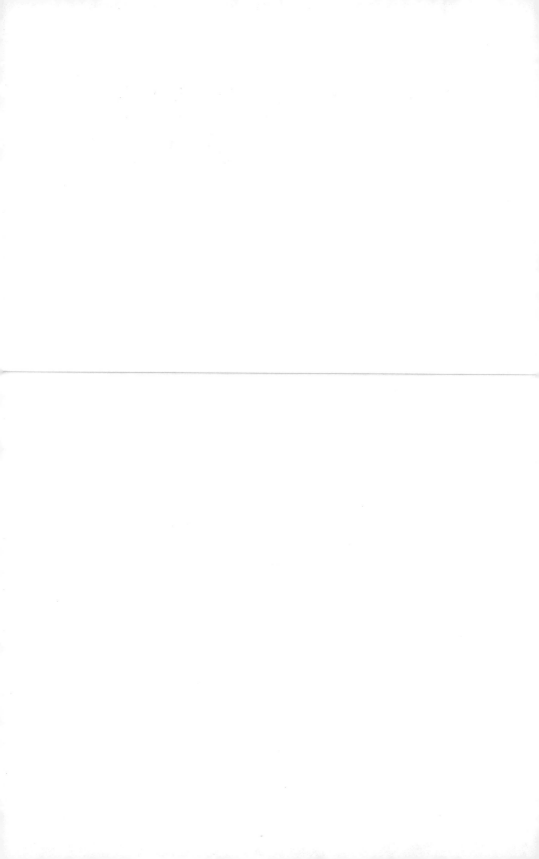

Executive Summary

ABSTRACT

In response to a request from Congress, the Institute of Medicine (IOM) convened a committee to conduct an analysis of the federal government's quality enhancement processes in six government programs—Medicare, Medicaid, the State Children's Health Insurance Program, the Department of Defense TRICARE and TRICARE for Life programs, the Veterans Health Administration program, and the Indian Health Services program. About one-third of Americans are beneficiaries of and the majority of health care providers participate in one or more of these programs.

The IOM committee encourages the federal government to take full advantage of its influential position to set the quality standard for the health care sector. Specifically, regulatory processes should be used to establish clinical data reporting requirements; purchasing strategies should provide rewards to providers who achieve higher levels of quality; health care delivery systems operated by public programs should serve as laboratories for the development of 21st-century care delivery models; and applied health services research should be expanded to accelerate the development of knowledge and tools in support of quality enhancement.

A strong quality infrastructure consisting of three components should be built. First, the Quality Interagency Coordinating Task Force, working with the private sector, should establish standardized performance measures to be applied in each of the government programs. Second, Congress and each of the six government programs should provide financial support and other incentives to providers to facilitate the development of information technology infrastructures. Finally, each government program should make quality reports available in the public domain for use by consumers, health care professionals, accreditation and certification bodies, and other stakeholders.

1

The U.S. health care sector faces serious safety, quality, coverage, and cost challenges. The United States spends much more per capita ($4,637 in 2000) on health care than any other country (Reinhardt et al., 2002), yet Americans cannot count on receiving care that is safe and effective (Institute of Medicine, 1999; Leatherman and McCarthy, 2002). While health care represents 13 percent of the U.S. gross domestic product—about $1.3 trillion annually (Levit et al., 2002)—one in seven Americans do not even have health insurance, and there are disturbing disparities in care for certain racial and ethnic subgroups (Institute of Medicine, 2002b, 2002c).

A major redesign of the health care sector is needed (Institute of Medicine, 2001). This redesign can occur only in an environment that fosters and rewards improvement. The Institute of Medicine's (IOM) 2001 report *Crossing the Quality Chasm: A New Health System for the 21st Century* calls for a "new environment for care" with payment incentives to encourage and reward innovation, precise streams of accountability and measurement reflecting quality achievements, and information and support to help engage consumers in understanding and interpreting information on quality and safety.

In this context, Congress asked the IOM to examine the federal government's quality enhancement processes (the Healthcare Research and Quality Act of 1999, Public Law 106-129) in six government programs—Medicare, Medicaid, the State Children's Health Insurance Program (SCHIP), the Department of Defense TRICARE and TRICARE for Life programs (DOD TRICARE), the Veterans Health Administration (VHA) program, and the Indian Health Service (IHS) program (see Table ES-1).

OVERVIEW OF CURRENT
QUALITY ENHANCEMENT PROCESSES

Each of the six programs reviewed for this study has both minimum participatory standards for providers and ongoing performance assessment activities.

Minimum participatory standards for institutional providers and clinicians are intended to ensure that program participants possess minimal levels of competence and comply with health and safety requirements. For institutions, the standards include physical safety and sanitation requirements and organizational requirements that enable specific activities such as governance, credentialing of medical staff, and quality improvement processes. For clinicians, the standards generally require compliance with the licensing laws of at least one state. Minimum participation standards reflect a good deal of consistency among programs.

Across all six government programs, there has been a proliferation of

TABLE ES-1 Government Health Care Programs in Fiscal Year 2001

Program	Beneficiaries	Expenditures
Medicare	40 million aged and disabled beneficiaries	$242.4 billion
Medicaid	42.3 million low-income persons; mostly children, pregnant women, disabled, and aged	$227.9 billion (joint federal and state)
SCHIP	4.6 million low-income children	$4.6 billion (joint federal and state)
VHA	4.0 million veterans	$20.9 billion
DOD TRICARE	8.4 million active-duty military personnel and their families and military retirees	$14.2 billion
IHS	1.4 million American Indians and Alaska Natives	$2.6 billion
TOTAL	About 100 million people [a]	$512.6 billion

[a]This estimate does not adjust for those beneficiaries who are eligible for more than one government program.
SOURCES: Department of Health and Human Services, 2002; Paisano, 2002; Veterans Administration, 2001; Williams, 2002.

performance assessment activities focused on the measurement of specific aspects of care processes and patient outcomes. The Medicare program relies mainly on external reviews of provider performance by quality improvement organizations (QIOs). In recent years, the Centers for Medicare and Medicaid Services (CMS) has required certain providers participating in Medicare—including Medicare+Choice plans, End Stage Renal Disease Networks, and, most recently, nursing homes—to comply with standardized quality reporting requirements. Federal law pertaining to the Medicaid program requires that states establish a plan for reviewing the appropriateness and quality of care, and most states contract with QIOs to carry out these reviews (Verdier and Dodge, 2002). The VHA, DOD TRICARE, and IHS programs all have incorporated a wealth of performance measurement activities into their health care delivery processes; in some instances, these programs also have contracts with external review organizations to review selected aspects of quality.

OPPORTUNITIES FOR IMPROVEMENT

A critical first step in addressing the nation's serious health care safety and quality concerns is the establishment of valid and reliable measurement systems that can be used to assess the degree to which care processes are consistent with the clinical knowledge base and patients are achieving desired outcomes. Clinical quality measurement provides the essential foundation for both quality improvement and accountability.

Although the quality enhancement processes of the major government programs are moving in a reasonably consistent and appropriate direction, the current set of activities has not closed the quality gap and is unlikely to do so in the future unless changes are made. This is the case for a number of reasons:

1. *A lack of consistency in performance measurement requirements both across and within individual government programs.* In Medicare and Medicaid performance measurement requirements are quite extensive for managed care plans and to a lesser degree for hospitals. On the other hand, performance measurement requirements are minimal or nonexistent for noninstitutional providers under fee-for-service arrangements, which still account for the majority of health care services. States have considerable latitude in the way they choose to define, implement, and enforce quality review in Medicaid and SCHIP programs; not surprisingly, the level and degree of external review activity vary widely among and within state programs.

2. *The absence of standardized performance measures, resulting in an unnecessary burden on providers and diminished usefulness of quality information.* Although some government programs have undertaken efforts to adopt standardized measures, these represent isolated success stories. The majority of performance measurement activities being carried out by the major government health care programs are neither standardized nor evenly applied across the programs. For private-sector providers, who typically participate in more than one government health care program, such variability in measures results in an excessive administrative burden.

3. *The lack of a conceptual framework to guide the selection of performance measures, resulting in a patchwork of measurement projects.* What generally appears to be missing is a clear conceptual framework with criteria that can guide the selection of individual measures to help maximize the health of the population being served.

4. *A lack of computerized clinical data.* VHA and DOD have made noteworthy strides in establishing a clinical information infrastructure, and the ability of their programs to measure and improve quality through continuous feedback and the application of computerized decision sup-

port systems is superior to what is typically found in the private sector. On the other hand, Medicare, Medicaid, SCHIP, and DOD TRICARE contracted health services must rely to a great extent on 20th-century measurement technology (e.g., abstraction of samples of medical records and culling of information from administrative datasets).

5. *The lack of a strong commitment to transparency and the availability of comparative quality data in the public domain.* Key stakeholders in each of the government programs—beneficiaries, providers, accrediting and certifying entities, regulators, and purchasers—have little useful information that can guide efforts to address the serious safety and quality shortcomings of the health care sector.

6. *The absence of a systematic approach for assessing the impact of quality enhancement activities.* Most minimum-participatory standards have been in place for a very long time, with little effort having been made to evaluate their effectiveness and the costs of compliance.

THE NEED FOR FEDERAL LEADERSHIP NOW

The federal government has a fiduciary responsibility to taxpayers and beneficiaries to ensure that the more than $500 billion invested annually in the six government programs is used wisely. Given the current deficiencies in health care safety and quality, it is clear that the federal government should be doing much more.

No other stakeholder has the federal government's ability to produce fundamental change throughout the health care sector. Absent strong federal leadership in addressing safety and quality concerns, progress will continue to be slow.

RECOMMENDATION 1: The federal government should assume a strong leadership position in driving the health care sector to improve the safety and quality of health care services provided to the approximately 100 million beneficiaries of the six major government health care programs. Given the leverage of the federal government, this leadership will result in improvements in the safety and quality of health care provided to all Americans.

This does not mean that the federal government should act alone. Indeed, its efforts will be far more effective if carried out in close collaboration with health care leadership from the private sector.

Each of the six government programs is already redesigning its quality enhancement processes. Unless there is more deliberate coordination, opportunities to achieve substantial gains in quality will be lost. The IOM committee that conducted this study encourages the leadership of the various government health care programs to ensure that their quality enhancement processes adhere to the following guiding principles:

1. *Government health care programs should establish consistent quality expectations and requirements and apply them fairly and equitably to all financing and delivery options within a program.*

2. *Government health care programs should promote and encourage providers to strive for excellence by providing financial and other rewards and public recognition to providers who achieve superior levels of quality.*

3. *Government health care programs should actively collaborate with each other and private-sector quality enhancement organizations with regard to all aspects of quality enhancement—including use of standardized measures and sharing of data—where doing so will likely result in greater gains in quality or reduced provider burden.*

4. *Government health care programs should encourage and enable active consumer participation in efforts to enhance quality through such means as the following:*

     a. *Raising consumer awareness of the magnitude of quality and safety shortcomings and the means of addressing these problems*

     b. *Seeking consumer input into the design and evaluation of quality enhancement processes*

     c. *Including patient assessments of quality and service in the portfolio of performance measures*

     d. *Providing patients with health information necessary to evaluate treatment options and participate in care management*

     e. *Providing consumers with comparative performance data on providers and health plans*

4. *Government health care programs, in collaboration with the Agency for Healthcare Research and Quality (AHRQ), should pursue a rich agenda of applied research and demonstrations focusing on tools, techniques, and approaches to quality enhancement.*

THE FEDERAL GOVERNMENT'S UNIQUE POSITION

In providing leadership to effect the needed changes in health care, the federal government should take full advantage of its unique position as a regulator; purchaser; health care provider; and sponsor of research, education, and training. As *regulator*, the federal government sets the standards for minimally acceptable performance. As the largest *purchaser* of health care services, the federal government institutes payment policies that determine the financial rewards or penalties that either spur or stifle innovations aimed at improving safety and quality. As a direct *provider* of health care services to veterans, military personnel and their families, and

Native Americans, the federal government can serve as a model for all aspects of health care organization and delivery. The federal government also provides support for applied health services research, much of which directly enhances the government's ability to carry out effectively its roles as regulator, purchaser, and health care provider.

In the government health care programs that provide care through the private sector—Medicare, Medicaid, SCHIP, and to some degree DOD TRICARE—the federal government has relied primarily on regulatory approaches to promote quality. Regulatory approaches are best suited to establishing a "floor" that protects beneficiaries from providers lacking basic competencies. When it comes to encouraging providers to pursue higher standards of excellence, the regulatory approach is a blunt tool that generally fails to differentiate among grades of quality.

Purchasing strategies are aimed at raising the quality of care offered by the majority of providers. Such strategies include the provision of financial and other rewards (e.g., higher fees, Diagnosis Related Group [DRG] payments, or bonuses) to providers and health plans achieving high levels of quality. The disclosure of comparative performance data on providers and health plans draws attention to best practices in the hope of driving patient volume to the higher-quality performers, and spurring action on the part of poor and average performers to enhance their knowledge and skills or limit their scope of practice. The public disclosure of quality and safety information may also encourage professional societies, board certifying and accrediting entities, and other leadership organizations to take action to achieve broader adherence to defined standards of care.

In its provider role, the federal government assumes all the responsibilities of ownership of health care institutions, employment of the health care workforce, and management and operation of comprehensive delivery systems. In this capacity, it has an opportunity to serve as a laboratory for the testing of new financing, delivery, and information dissemination models while experimenting with various quality measurement and improvement strategies. The three government programs that provide services directly—the VHA, DOD TRICARE, and IHS programs—have led the way in building clinical information systems to support care delivery, quality improvement, surveillance and monitoring, and many other applications. Since taxpayer dollars have financed the development of these systems, more should be done to facilitate their application in other parts of the health care system.

As a major sponsor of applied health services research, the federal government provides support for the development of knowledge and the creation of tools needed to carry out more effectively the roles of regulator, purchaser, and health care provider. Through AHRQ and other applied research programs sponsored by VHA, the National Institutes of Health, and the Centers for Disease Control and Prevention, the federal government can and has assisted in the development of quality measures, survey instruments, and public reporting tools. The federal government also supports applied health services research that addresses many of the broader health care financing and delivery issues whose resolution is important to creating an environment that supports quality.

> **RECOMMENDATION 2: The federal government should take maximal advantage of its unique position as regulator, health care purchaser, health care provider, and sponsor of applied health services research to set quality standards for the health care sector. Specifically:**
>
> **a. Regulatory processes should be used to establish clinical data reporting requirements applicable to all six major government health care programs.**
>
> **b. All six major government health care programs should vigorously pursue purchasing strategies that encourage the adoption of best practices through the release of public-domain comparative quality data and the provision of financial and other rewards to providers that achieve high levels of quality.**
>
> **c. Not only should health care delivery systems operated by the public programs continue to serve as laboratories for the development of innovative 21st-century care delivery models, but much greater emphasis should be placed on the dissemination of findings and, in the case of information technology, the creation of public-domain products.**
>
> **d. Applied health services research should be expanded and should emphasize the development of knowledge, tools, and strategies that can support quality enhancement in a wide variety of settings.**

Congress should provide the appropriate direction, enabling authority, and resources to the government health care programs for carrying out this mandate.

THE TRANSFORMATION OF QUALITY ENHANCEMENT

At present, the federal government is seriously hampered in performing its purchasing, regulatory, and provider functions by a lack of information on clinical quality—the degree to which the care received by beneficiaries is consistent with the science base (i.e., effective) and provided in a technically competent fashion (i.e., safe).

Variability in performance measures and activities across and within government programs limits the ability to draw comparisons; imposes an unnecessary burden on providers that participate in multiple programs; and makes it difficult to obtain a complete picture of the quality of care for beneficiaries, especially dual eligibles. The uneven application of performance measurement requirements across various delivery sites and beneficiary populations on the part of some government programs fails to provide equitable protections to all program beneficiaries. Moreover, providers do not receive strong, consistent signals as to where quality improvement is needed. There is also a paucity of comparative quality data available in the public domain for use by other stakeholders, including consumers, providers, professional associations, purchasers, and private accrediting and certifying entities.

> **RECOMMENDATION 3: Congress should direct the Secretaries of the Department of Health and Human Services, Department of Defense, and Department of Veterans Affairs to work together to establish standardized performance measures across the government programs, as well as public reporting requirements for clinicians, institutional providers, and health plans in each program. These requirements should be implemented for all six major government health care programs and should be applied fairly and equitably across various financing and delivery options within those programs. The standardized measurement and reporting activities should replace the many performance measurement activities currently under way in the various government programs.**

The proposed changes in quality enhancement processes will necessitate substantial reorientation and operational change within all three government branches, so leadership and support will be necessary from the highest levels of the Department of Health and Human Services (DHHS), DOD, and VHA. At the same time, there should be a focal point for coordination and accountability. Congress should consider directing the Secretary of Health and Human Services to assume a lead role in producing an annual progress report detailing the collaborative and individual efforts of the various government programs to redesign their quality enhancement processes.

To achieve the objective of this recommendation, a stronger quality infrastructure consisting of three major components—standardized performance measures, computerized clinical information, and comparative quality reporting in the public domain—must be developed.

Standardized Performance Measures

In developing a menu of standardized performance measures for health care quality, the federal government should not reinvent the wheel. Rather, it should build on work already under way in both the private and public sectors to establish a common conceptual framework for performance measurement and reporting. In 2003, DHHS will be releasing the first National Healthcare Quality Report, which will include measures relevant to six national quality aims recommended by the IOM in an earlier report—safety, effectiveness, patient-centeredness, timeliness, efficiency, and equity (Institute of Medicine, 2001). The National Healthcare Quality Report will also focus on priority health areas—common chronic conditions and health care needs of the population (Institute of Medicine, 2002a). Use of a common conceptual framework, common terminology, and, whenever possible, standardized measures for reporting at all levels—national, regional, and provider-specific—will facilitate understanding and action on the part of all stakeholders and reduce the burden of compliance.

The Quality Interagency Coordination Task Force (QuIC) (or some similar interdepartmental structure) should play a pivotal role in the establishment of standardized performance measures. The QuIC was created in 1998 to provide coordination across federal agencies involved in regulating, purchasing, providing, and studying health care services. Its membership already includes representatives of CMS, AHRQ, VHA, DOD, IHS, and other federal programs, and could be expanded to include representatives from state Medicaid and SCHIP programs and consumers. The QuIC should collaborate with such private-sector groups as the National Quality Forum (NQF), the Leapfrog Group, the National Committee for Quality Assurance (NCQA), the Joint Commission on Accreditation of Healthcare Organizations (JCAHO), and the Foundation for Accountability (FAACT) in the development of performance measures to avoid duplication of effort and conflict with the activities of these groups. NQF, in particular, was established in 1999 to convene public- and private-sector stakeholders to seek consensus around standardized measures (Miller and Leatherman, 1999), and CMS has worked collaboratively with NQF to develop standardized measures in particular areas (National Quality Forum, 2000).

RECOMMENDATION 4: The QuIC should promulgate standardized sets of performance measures for 5 common health conditions in fiscal year (FY) 2003 and another 10 sets in FY 2004.

a. Each government health care program should pilot test the first 5 sets of measures between FY 2003 and FY 2005 in a limited num-

ber of sites. These pilot tests should include the collection of patient-level data and the public release of comparative performance reports.

b. All six government programs should prepare for full implementation of the 15-set performance measurement and reporting system by FY 2008. The government health care programs that provide services through the private sector (i.e., Medicare, Medicaid, SCHIP, and portions of DOD TRICARE) should inform participating providers that submission of the audited patient-level data necessary for performance measurement will be required for continued participation in FY 2007. The government health care programs that provide services directly (i.e., VHA, the remainder of DOD TRICARE, and IHS) should begin work immediately to ensure that they have the information technology capabilities to produce the necessary data.

Although there should be a common menu of standardized performance measures, not all measures would have to be implemented in all government programs. Each program would select the subset of measures that corresponded to its beneficiaries' clinical needs.

Computerized Clinical Data

Although it may be feasible in the short run for providers to produce the patient-level data needed for performance measurement through record abstraction or special data collection instruments, it will not always be possible to rely upon such approaches as the menu of measures expands—nor should it be. Computerized clinical data and decision support systems are a prerequisite for the safe provision of quality care (Institute of Medicine, 2001). The potential benefits of computerized clinical data and decision support have long been recognized (Institute of Medicine, 1997), but only recently has the evidence base emerged to substantiate these expectations (Balas et al., 2000; Bates et al., 1999; Classen et al., 1997; Leapfrog Group, 2000; Raymond and Dold, 2002; Shea et al., 1996).

In general, the health care delivery sector has lagged behind other industries in adopting and making innovative use of information technology. This is especially true for the private sector, and less so for the public-sector delivery systems of VHA and DOD.

The federal government has an important role to play in offering financial incentives to health care providers. It was beyond the scope of this study to develop estimates of the resources required to build the necessary information technology infrastructure, but the need for such support should not be underestimated. In the absence of adequate assistance, it will not be possible for providers to adhere to the ambitious timetable for quality enhancement proposed in this report.

RECOMMENDATION 5: The federal government should take steps immediately to encourage and facilitate the development of the information technology infrastructure that is critical to health care quality and safety enhancement, as well as to many of the nation's other priorities, such as bioterrorism surveillance, public health, and research. Specifically:

a. Congress should consider potential options to facilitate rapid development of a national health information infrastructure, including tax credits, subsidized loans, and grants.

b. Government health care programs that deliver services through the private sector (Medicare, Medicaid, SCHIP, and a portion of DOD TRICARE) should adopt both market-based and regulatory options to encourage investment in information technology. Such options might include enhanced or more rapid payments to providers capable of submitting computerized clinical data, a requirement for certain information technology capabilities as a condition of participation, and direct grants.

c. VHA, DOD, and IHS should continue implementing clinical and administrative information systems that enable the retrieval of clinical information across their programs and can communicate directly with each other. Whenever possible, the software and intellectual property developed by these three government programs should rely on Web-based language and architecture and be made available in the public domain.

In addition to offering financial incentives to providers, the federal government should play a stronger role in the establishment of national standards for the collection, coding, and classification of clinical and other health care data (National Committee on Vital and Health Statistics, 2001). Some degree of technical assistance may also be required, especially for safety net providers.

Comparative Quality Reporting

There are many potential uses of comparative quality data. First, providers and care systems that are working to achieve continuous improvement might use the data for benchmarking purposes and to inform decisions regarding referral of patients to specialists and hospitals. Second, patients and group purchasers might access the data when choosing health plans or providers. Third, professional groups, including board certification entities such as the American Board of Medical Specialties and its member boards, might be able to use the data to identify best practices and to assist in making credentialing decisions. Fourth, private accreditation organizations, such as NCQA and JCAHO, and public regulatory programs might use the data in their efforts to assess provider compliance with requirements and to provide information to the public. Fifth, the data will likely be useful to states, communities, and public health groups as a tool for identifying gaps in quality and monitoring the impact of community-wide efforts to close these gaps.

RECOMMENDATION 6: Starting in FY 2008, each government health care program should make comparative quality reports and data available in the public domain. The programs should provide for access to these reports and data in ways that meet the needs of various users, provided that patient privacy is protected.

Many private-sector stakeholders, such as accreditors and purchasers, already impose quality reporting requirements on providers. The committee encourages the government programs to work with these groups on the design, pilot testing, and rollout of the above reports. Doing so will increase the likelihood that these stakeholders will incorporate the standardized measures and reports into their processes, thus further reducing administrative burden.

A mechanism should be established for pooling data from each of the government health care programs. Pooled data would facilitate benchmarking across a wide variety of financing and delivery arrangements, population subgroups, and geographic areas. The availability of such data would also allow for the analysis of more complete care patterns for beneficiaries receiving services under more than one government program.

RECOMMENDATION 7: The government health care programs, working with AHRQ, should establish a mechanism for pooling performance measurement data across programs in a data repository. Contributions of data from private-sector insurance programs should be encouraged provided such data meet certain standards for validity and reliability. Consumers, health care professionals, planners, purchasers, regulators, public health officials, researchers, and others should be afforded access to the repository, provided that patient privacy is protected.

The desirability of providing broad access to the repository by many stakeholders must be balanced by the need to both protect patient privacy and minimize harmful, unintended consequences of public disclosure. Patient-level data included in the repository should be deidentified to prevent individual patient identification, and any users violating data access policies should be subject to severe penalties.

NEED FOR APPLIED HEALTH SERVICES RESEARCH

Steps should be taken to ensure that the health services research agendas developed by the various government programs are complementary, address the needs of the populations served, and advance the capabilities of quality enhancement processes to promote excellence. Given its mission to coordinate the implementation of quality enhancement processes among the six government programs and its representative membership, the QuIC is well positioned to serve as the coordinating entity through which programs would provide input on the research and development agenda. AHRQ should staff the QuIC and provide the organizational locus of QuIC research activity.

> **RECOMMENDATION 8: The six government health care programs should work together to develop a comprehensive health services research agenda that will support the quality enhancement processes of all programs. The QuIC (or some similar interdepartmental structure with representation from each of the government health care programs and AHRQ) should be provided the authority and resources needed to carry out this responsibility. The agenda for FY 2003–2005 should support the following:**
>
> **a. Establishment of core sets of standardized performance measures**
>
> **b. Ongoing evaluation of the impact of the use of standardized performance measurement and reporting by the six major government health care programs**
>
> **c. Development and evaluation of specific strategies that can be used to improve the federal government's capability to leverage its purchaser, regulator, and provider roles to enhance quality**
>
> **d. Monitoring of national progress in meeting the six national quality aims (safety, effectiveness, patient-centeredness, timeliness, efficiency, and equity)**

Formulation of the federal health services research agenda should address the immediate need of the QuIC to establish a core set of standardized performance measures. Efforts should be made to address methodological issues, especially those related to the assessment of quality at the small group or individual clinician level. Attention should also be focused on the design and pilot testing of alternative reporting formats tailored to the needs of various users.

Evaluation of the impact of standardized performance measurement and reporting efforts should include assessment of the associated reduction in burden, as well as identification of opportunities for further eliminating redundancy and ineffective regulatory requirements. As discussed above, current quality enhancement processes fall into two categories: minimum participatory requirements and performance assessment. The specific performance measurement activities in each of the government programs that have been superceded by standardized measurement and reporting activities should be documented. Once a robust quality infrastructure has been established, an assessment should be conducted to determine whether some minimum participatory standards might be eliminated.

GETTING FROM HERE TO THERE

The committee has formulated a very rigorous implementation strategy that calls for the release of an initial set of comparative performance reports for a limited set of standardized measures in 3 years and a fully operational process in 6 years (see Figure ES-1). Specifically, the QuIC would identify standardized performance measure sets for 5 priority areas in FY 2003 and for 10 more in FY 2004.

Pilot testing of the first 5 sets of measures would begin immediately, with the objective of each government program's release of comparative performance reports (probably for a few selected geographic areas) for this limited number of measures in FY 2005. Starting in FY 2007, providers participating in the government programs that offer services through the private sector would be required to submit performance data as a condition of participation. Installation of compatible information technology systems across VHA, DOD, and IHS should be completed in 2006 to enable better evaluation of quality of care in government-operated health programs. In FY 2008, each government health care program should publicly release a comprehensive set of comparative quality reports for all 15 priority areas and all provider types. A vigorous applied research and demonstration capability will be necessary throughout this period, starting in FY 2003 with the development of an agenda to address key measurement and methodological issues, design of the pilot test, conduct of periodic evaluations, and preparation of a final evaluation upon completion of the 6-year implementation period.

The committee realizes this is an ambitious agenda. It does not, however, represent a radical departure from the status quo, but rather a rapid scaling up of the most promising, cutting-edge quality enhancement projects currently under way. It is important not to underestimate the challenges of progressing from what are essentially promising pilot

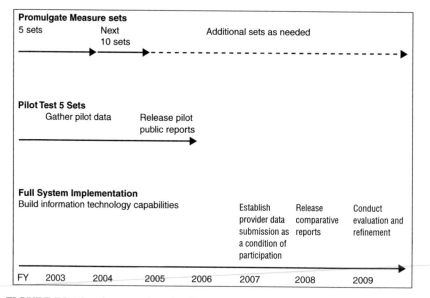

FIGURE ES-1 Implementation timeline.

projects to widespread adoption of a new strategic direction and major redesign of the quality enhancement processes of the six government programs. The committee has identified four factors that will be critical to the success of this endeavor.

First, to avoid major delays in moving forward, it would be wise to identify potential legal and regulatory barriers early on and determine how best to address these barriers expeditiously. For example, does the emphasis on public reporting of deidentified data raise any concerns with regard to the confidentiality and security provisions of the Health Insurance Portability and Accountability Act? Will additional enabling authority be required for CMS to move forward with demonstration projects that provide financial rewards to providers who achieve exemplary performance?

Second, conscious and careful redesign of the quality enhancement processes of each of the major government programs will be necessary. The standardized quality measurement and reporting activities proposed in this report are not intended to represent another layer of government oversight, but rather to replace the patchwork of quality measurement activities and projects currently under way. Nowhere will these changes be more significant than in the Medicare, Medicaid, and SCHIP programs, which rely on a mix of public- and private-sector external review entities, and in some cases on a blend of federal and state requirements and initiatives.

The backbone of Medicare's external quality review processes is the QIOs. The QIOs are engaged in some projects that employ common measures and methodologies across most or all states, and this approach is increasingly becoming the norm. Much of the quality-related data used by QIOs is abstracted from samples of paper medical records or culled from claims data—methods that will likely become obsolete as computerized patient-level data become more readily available. QIOs have limited experience in public reporting, although sizable resources are earmarked for this function in their Seventh Scope of Work. Contractual, cultural, organizational, and programmatic modifications will be required for the QIO program to continue playing a central role in the quality enhancement processes of Medicare and other government health care programs.

The challenges for state Medicaid and SCHIP programs will also be significant. Under the proposed restructuring, states will be asked to relinquish some flexibility and to work in partnership with each other and federal government representatives from the six programs to agree upon standardized performance measurement sets and to apply these standardized measures across their Medicaid and SCHIP programs. States have already worked with CMS, each other, and NCQA on the development of the Health Plan Employer Data and Information Set (HEDIS) standardized measures adapted for state Medicaid programs, and these measures are being used for health plans with a good deal of uniformity in adoption and application. What is being sought here is a much stronger commitment to standardized measurement and reporting.

Third, strong support from the appropriate authorization and appropriations committees of Congress will be critical to success. Federal financial assistance to providers will be essential to establishing the necessary information technology infrastructure. AHRQ will require additional funds to provide adequate support to the QuIC for the establishment and maintenance of the menu of standardized measures, the design and pilot testing of reporting formats, the establishment and operation of the repository of pooled data, and the conduct of periodic evaluations of the impact of the new quality enhancement strategies. Lastly, some initial support for each of the government programs will also be needed so they can redesign their current oversight processes and establish the capacities required to receive and process the necessary clinical data and produce reports.

Fourth, the federal and state governments should immediately begin working in partnership with health care leaders, including representatives of consumer groups, the health professions, and health care organizations. It will be challenging to transform the current quality enhancement processes of the government programs into standardized quality reporting structures that are transparent and contribute to an environment rich in comparative quality information. This transformation will be much smoother if the QuIC and CMS, in particular, establish strong partnerships with stakeholders. Consumers, participating providers, and health plans should receive complete and timely information—there should be no surprises. Special efforts should be made early on to secure the support of leaders from the medical, nursing, and other health professions, and to build on the basic tenets of professionalism (American Board of Internal Medicine et al., 2002). The government health care programs should move expeditiously to address all legitimate questions and concerns about their quality enhancement processes, including the reliability and validity of information, measures, and data. All parties should recognize that problems will be encountered along the way with data, measures, and reports, necessitating continuous improvement and refinement. There must also be rewards and benefits for providers taking part in these efforts in the form of reduced regulatory burden, feedback of information useful for quality improvement, and public recognition and financial rewards for exemplary performance.

REFERENCES

American Board of Internal Medicine, ACP-ASIM Foundation, and European Federation of Internal Medicine. 2002. Medical professionalism in the new millennium: a physician charter. *Ann Intern Med* 136 (3).

Balas, E. A., S. Weingarten, C. T. Garb, D. Blumenthal, S. A. Boren, and G. D. Brown. 2000. Improving preventive care by prompting physicians. *Arch Intern Med* 160 (3):301-8.

Bates, D. W., J. M. Teich, J. Lee, D. Seger, G. J. Kuperman, N. Ma'Luf, D. Boyle, and L. Leape. 1999. The impact of computerized physician order entry on medication error prevention. *J Am Med Inform Assoc* 6 (4):313-21.

Classen, D. C., S. L. Pestrotnik, R. S. Evans, et al. 1997. Adverse drug events in hospitalized patients. *JAMA* 277 (4):301-6.

Department of Health and Human Services. 2002. *2002 CMS Statistics. CMS Publication No. 03437.* Baltimore MD: U.S. Department of Health and Human Services.

Institute of Medicine. 1997. *The Computer-Based Patient Record: An Essential Technology for Health Care.* Washington DC: National Academy Press.

———. 1999. *To Err Is Human: Building a Safer Health System.* Washington DC: National Academy Press.

———. 2001. *Crossing the Quality Chasm: A New Health System for the 21st Century.* Washington DC: National Academy Press.

———. 2002a. *Priority Areas for National Action: Transforming Health Care Quality.* Washington DC: National Academy Press.

———. 2002b. *Unequal Treatment: Confronting Racial and Ethnic Disparities in Health Care.* B. Smedley, A. Stith, and A. Nelson, eds. Washington DC: National Academy Press.

———. 2002c. *Care Without Coverage.* Washington DC: National Academy Press.

Leapfrog Group. 2000. "Fact Sheet: Computer Physician Order Entry (CPOE)." Online. Available at http://www.leapfroggroup.org/FactSheets/CPOE_FactSheet.pdf [accessed May 16, 2002].

Leatherman, S., and D. McCarthy. 2002. *Quality of Health in the United States: A Chartbook.* New York NY: The Commonwealth Fund.

Levit, K., C. Smith, C. Cowan, et al. 2002. Inflation spurs health spending in 2000. *Health Aff (Millwood)* 21 (1):172-81.

Miller, T., and S. Leatherman. 1999. The National Quality Forum: a "me-too" or a breakthrough in quality measurement and reporting? *Health Aff (Millwood)* 18 (6):233-7.

National Committee on Vital and Health Statistics. 2001. "Information for Health: A Strategy for Building the National Health Information Infrastructure." Online. Available at http://ncvhs.hhs.gov/nhiilayo.pdf [accessed May 14, 2002].

National Quality Forum. 2000. NQF project brief: Measuring serious, avoidable adverse events in hospital care. *National Forum for Health Care Quality Measurement and Reporting.*

Paisano, E. (IHS). 1 July 2002. IHS total expenditure data. Personal communication to Barbara Smith.

Raymond, B., and C. Dold. 2002. *Clinical Information Systems: Achieving the Vision.* Oakland CA: Kaiser Permanente for Health Policy.

Reinhardt, U. E., P. S. Hussey, and G. F. Anderson. 2002. Cross-national comparisons of health systems using OECD data, 1999. *Health Aff (Millwood)* 21 (3):169-81.

Shea, S., W. DuMouchel, and L. Bahamonde. 1996. A meta-analysis of 16 randomized controlled trials to evaluate computer-based clinical reminder systems for preventive care in the ambulatory setting. *J Am Med Inform Assoc* 3 (6): 399-409.

Verdier, J., and R. Dodge. 2002. *Other Data Sources and Uses, Working Paper in the Informed Purchasing Series.* Lawrenceville NJ: Center for Health Care Strategies.

Veterans Administration. 2001. "VA Budget Overview 2002." Online. Available at http://www.va.gov/pressrel/bdgtovrw_files/bdgtovrw.htm [accessed June 28, 2002].

Williams, T. (TMA) 2 July 2002. TRICARE total expenditure data. Personal communication to Barbara Smith.

1

Introduction

The provision of health care services to the diverse U.S. population represents one of the largest segments of the nation's economy—approximately one-seventh of its gross domestic product (Centers for Medicare and Medicaid Services, 2002). The government health care programs that are the focus of this report—Medicare, Medicaid, the State Children's Health Insurance Program (SCHIP), the Department of Defense TRICARE and TRICARE for Life programs (referred to collectively as DOD TRICARE), the Veterans Health Administration (VHA) program, and the Indian Health Service (IHS) program—account for over 40 percent of all health care expenditures in the United States. Consequently, the federal government has a central and pervasive role in shaping nearly all aspects of the health care sector, both public and private. A critical question is how the federal government can use this leverage to improve the quality of care for all Americans.

Quality of care can be defined as the degree to which health services for individuals and populations increase the likelihood of desired health outcomes and are consistent with current professional knowledge (Institute of Medicine, 1990).

STUDY PROCESS AND SCOPE

In 1999, Congress asked the Institute of Medicine (IOM) to convene a panel of experts to explore ways of enhancing the quality of care offered through government health care programs (the Healthcare Research and Quality Act of 1999, Public Law 106-129). Underlying the scope and intent of this study is the judgment that, by virtue of its breadth of involvement in health care regulation, purchasing, provision of services, and sponsorship of research and education, the federal government can and should have a significant influence on quality of care in all aspects of health care programs and services available to the American people, whether provided through a government health care program or not.

To carry out this study, the IOM established the Committee on Enhancing Federal Healthcare Quality Programs. The committee's mandate was to examine for each of the above six government programs those specific operational components whose function is to assure and improve the quality of care received by beneficiaries. The committee has chosen the term "quality enhancement processes" to represent the set of government activities encompassed by this function. Quality enhancement processes include, among other things, the following four components:

• Requirements directed at enhancing provider competencies, both for institutional providers and for members of the health professions
• Periodic or ongoing assessment of the quality of care, including measurement of the processes and outcomes of care
• Synthesis, analysis, and public reporting of quality assessment results by site or level of care
• Actions, based on the results of quality assessment activities, to effect changes in care processes or outcomes for defined categories of beneficiaries

Beyond these four components of quality enhancement processes, other aspects of care delivery systems have a substantial impact on the safety and quality of care provided to any beneficiary population. For example, the committee recognizes (and in Chapter 2 comments on) the impact of basic health care benefits, payment approaches, and program design and administrative issues on the processes and outcomes of care. Technological and scientific advances and education in the health professions are other important factors, but outside the scope of this report.

It is important to emphasize that the term "quality enhancement processes" implies much more than regulatory activities of governmental agencies. The federal government performs multiple roles in health care, including those of regulator; large group purchaser; health care provider;

and sponsor of health-related research, education, and training programs. The focus of this study is on quality enhancement activities of many kinds and at different levels intended to promote and enhance care processes and beneficiary outcomes. In addition, patient-centered (or consumer-centered) care has been identified as an essential element of quality health care (Institute of Medicine, 2001).

An investment in quality enhancement within the six major government health care programs will, in itself, make a difference in the lives of about 100 million Americans served by these programs. In carrying out its fiduciary responsibility, the federal government has the opportunity to serve as an important beacon of influence within the larger public and private health care sectors. For most health care providers, institutional and individual alike, the government health care programs constitute an important source of revenue. Quality improvement activities undertaken within these programs are likely to have an effect on overall quality of care that reaches beyond the programs themselves. Conversely, and perhaps more important, without the federal government's leadership, it will be difficult if not impossible to bring about the needed changes in a sector whose market signals are dominated by government-driven payment and regulation.

The principal objective of this report, then, is to provide guidance for improving the quality enhancement processes of government health care programs. There have been numerous expert reports examining the quality activities of individual programs (Department of Defense, 2001; MedPAC, 2002). This committee was presented with a different challenge: to examine the quality enhancement processes of all six major government health care programs. The committee's focus on multiple programs allows for the identification of opportunities to improve the effectiveness and efficiency of government quality oversight activities as a whole, as well as to make program-specific improvements. This focus also highlights the unique role the federal government can play in driving the redesign of the health care sector by leveraging its aggregate purchasing power.

STUDY CONTEXT

Quality of health care has become a significant concern of both public- and private-sector policy and program administration. For over two decades, there has been a steady flow of publications in leading peer-reviewed journals documenting widespread variability in quality (Jencks et al., 2000; Miller and Luft, 1993; Schuster et al., 1998). These gaps in quality are present for both capitated and fee-for-service insurance arrangements and across all geographic areas and health care delivery settings (Chassin and Galvin, 1998).

The convergence of a series of studies and reports beginning in 1998 has brought renewed urgency to the quality debate. These reports reveal widespread defects in the delivery of medical care that taken together "detract from the health, functioning, dignity, comfort, satisfaction, and resources of Americans" (Institute of Medicine, 2001, p. 2). According to the IOM's National Roundtable on Health Care Quality: "The burden of harm conveyed by the collective impact of all of our health care quality problems is staggering. . . . The challenge is to bring the full potential benefit of effective health care to all Americans while avoiding unneeded and harmful interventions and eliminating preventable complications of care. . . . Our present efforts resemble a team of engineers trying to break the sound barrier by tinkering with a Model T Ford" (Chassin and Galvin, 1998, p. 1004). The extent and impact of quality problems are confirmed in the report of the Advisory Commission on Consumer Protection and Quality in the Health Care Industry (Advisory Commission, 1998, p. 21): "[T]oday in America, there is no guarantee that any individual will receive high-quality care for any particular problem. The health care industry is plagued with overutilization . . . underutilization . . . and errors. . . . "

Results of studies of the treatment of specific diseases, such as cancers, indicate that serious quality problems emerge at virtually every stage of medical care (Institute of Medicine, 1999a). A lack of conformity with practice standards in the prevention, diagnosis, and treatment of disease is compounded by issues of basic patient safety in the delivery of care. Avoidable deaths due to medical errors exceed the number of deaths attributable to many leading causes of mortality, including AIDS, breast cancer, and motor vehicle crashes and injuries (Institute of Medicine, 1999b).

In its report *Crossing the Quality Chasm: A New Health System for the 21st Century*, the IOM (2001) calls for fundamental reform of the health care system directed at effecting substantial improvements to achieve six quality aims—safety, effectiveness, patient-centeredness, timeliness, efficiency, and equity. Achieving these aims will require changes at four levels: patient experiences, microsystems that deliver care (e.g., multidisciplinary team), health care organizations that house the microsystems (e.g., hospitals), and the environment (e.g., payment policies, regulatory framework) (Berwick, 2002).

This steady stream of analyses, pronouncements, and consensus perspectives has created a national climate within which it is now expected that responsible health care programs will be accountable for demonstrating that the services they provide not only meet minimal standards of care quality, but also achieve continuous improvement. Major public- and private-sector purchasers of care are demanding that steps be taken to improve the quality and safety of health care (Galvin, 2001). Because of the enormous influence of the six major government health care programs within the U.S. health care sector as a whole, the committee expects that these programs will attempt to address quality issues first, and most effectively.

ORGANIZATION OF THE REPORT

In this report, the committee responds to its charge by (a) describing the basic structure and beneficiary populations of the six major government health care programs, (b) documenting the activities of each of these programs with regard to the four principal components of quality enhancement identified above, and (c) offering recommendations for improving current quality enhancement processes.

Chapter 2 provides a description of each of the six government health care programs included in this study. It also reviews the broad trends affecting the needs and expectations of the programs' beneficiaries, as well as key program features other than quality enhancement processes that affect the quality of health care provided.

Chapter 3 reviews the various roles played by the federal government in the health care arena and examines how these roles can be leveraged and better coordinated to improve the quality enhancement processes and activities of the various government health care programs. In general, each of the programs has fairly well-developed regulatory processes for ensuring quality, including minimum standards of participation for providers and external quality review activities. The federal government has far less experience as a value-based purchaser, although there are several notable examples of small-scale efforts to encourage disclosure of comparative quality data and selectively purchase from or provide payment incentives to high-quality providers. Lastly, three of the government programs—DOD TRICARE and the VHA and IHS programs—own and operate extensive delivery systems that have to varying degrees incorporated quality improvement activities into their operations.

Chapter 4 proposes a national quality enhancement strategy focused on performance measurement that is based on standardized measures of clinical quality and patient perceptions of care—two areas that have in recent years received increased emphasis from all six programs. There are important similarities in the types of measures and approaches adopted by the various programs. The chapter stresses the need to develop standardized measures that address important priority areas and the importance of applying these standardized measures across all the government programs. Also examined are some of the methodological and operational challenges that must be confronted, including measurement at the level of individual physicians/groups and accountability for quality concerns that cut across providers and settings.

Chapter 5 calls for the federal government to work collaboratively with the private sector to establish processes for reporting, analyzing, and releasing performance measurement data. Under the national quality enhancement strategy recommended in this report, providers would submit performance data using standardized measures, and comparative performance data would be made available at various levels of detail to consumers, health care providers, purchasers, regulators, and other stakeholders. This chapter examines why a more sophisticated information infrastructure is critical both to the implementation of this quality enhancement strategy and to the achievement of threshold improvements in quality over the coming decade. It also explores the need for well-thought-out processes for the analysis, interpretation, and release of performance data.

Lastly, a strong health services research capability will be necessary to enable the establishment of standardized measures and public reporting functions across the various government health care programs. Chapter 6 provides an overview of current health services research activities related to quality oversight that are carried out by the various federal agencies. It also provides a rationale for a more coordinated process for development of a national health care quality research agenda.

Three appendices are also included. Appendix A is a list of the acronyms used in the report. Appendix B shows the performance measurement set that resulted from the Diabetes Quality Improvement Project, an effort to develop a standardized set of process and outcome measures for performance reporting related to the care of adults with diabetes. Finally, Appendix C presents a technical overview of the health information systems of VHA and DOD.

REFERENCES

Advisory Commission. 1998. Quality First: Better Health Care for All Americans. Final Report to the President of the United States. Washington DC: U.S. Government Printing Office.

Berwick, D. M. 2002. A user's manual for the IOM's "Quality Chasm Report": patients' experiences should be the fundamental source of the definition of "quality". Health Aff (Millwood) 21 (1):80-90.

Centers for Medicare and Medicaid Services. 2002. "National Health Expenditures Projections: 2001-2011." Online. Available at http://www.hcfa.gov/stats/nhe-proj/proj2001/default.htm [accessed March 20, 2002].

Chassin, M., and R. Galvin. 1998. The urgent need to improve health care quality: Institute of Medicine National Roundtable on Quality. JAMA 280 (11):1000-05.

Department of Defense. 2001. "Healthcare Quality Initiatives Review Panel (HQIRP) Report." Online. Available at http://www.tricare.osd.mil/downloads/FinalReport123.pdf [accessed June 26, 2002].

Galvin, R. 2001. The business case for quality. *Health Aff (Millwood)* 20 (6):57-58.

Institute of Medicine. 1990. *Medicare: A Strategy for Quality Assurance.* Volume I. Washington DC: National Academy Press.

———. 1999a. *Ensuring Quality Cancer Care.* Washington DC: National Academy Press.

———. 1999b. *To Err Is Human: Building a Safer Health System.* Washington DC: National Academy Press.

———. 2001. *Crossing the Quality Chasm: A New Health System for the 21st Century.* Washington DC: National Academy Press.

Jencks, S. F., T. Cuerdon, D. R. Burwen, B. Fleming, P. M. Houck, A. E. Kussmaul, D. S. Nilasena, D. L. Ordin, and D. R. Arday. 2000. Quality of medical care delivered to Medicare beneficiaries: A profile at state and national levels. *JAMA* 284 (13):1670-76.

MedPAC. 2002. "Report to Congress: Applying Quality Improvement Standards in Medicare." Online. Available at http://www.medpac.gov/publications/congressional_reports/jan2002_QualityImprovement.pdf [accessed Oct. 2, 2002].

Miller, R., and H. Luft. 1993. Managed care: past evidence and potential trends. *Front Health Serv Manage* 9 (3):3-37.

Schuster, M. A., E. A. McGlynn, and R. H. Brook. 1998. How good is the quality of health care in the United States? *Milbank Q* 76 (4):517-63.

2

Overview of the Government Health Care Programs

SUMMARY OF CHAPTER RECOMMENDATIONS

The six major government health care programs—Medicare, Medicaid, the State Children's Health Insurance Program (SCHIP), the Department of Defense TRICARE and TRICARE for Life programs (DOD TRICARE), the Veterans Health Administration (VHA) program, and the Indian Health Service (IHS) program—provide health care services to about one-third of Americans. The federal government has a responsibility to ensure that the more than $500 billion invested annually in these programs is used wisely to reduce the burden of illness, injury, and disability and to improve the health and functioning of the population. It is imperative that the federal government exercise strong leadership in addressing serious shortcomings in the safety and quality of health care in the United States.

RECOMMENDATION 1: The federal government should assume a strong leadership position in driving the health care sector to improve the safety and quality of health care services provided to the approximately 100 million beneficiaries of the six major government health care programs. Given the leverage of the federal government, this leadership will result in improvements in the safety and quality of health care provided to all Americans.

The six major government health care programs serve older persons, persons with disabilities, low-income mothers and children, veterans, active-duty military personnel and their dependents, and Native Americans. Three of these programs—Medicare, Medicaid, and the State Children's Health Insurance Program (SCHIP)—were devised for groups for whom the health care market has historically failed to work because of their high health care needs and low socioeconomic status. The remaining three programs—DOD TRICARE, VHA, and IHS—serve particular populations with whom the federal government has a special relationship, respectively, military personnel and their dependents, veterans, and Native Americans.

Many millions of Americans receive services through multiple government programs simultaneously. Low-income Medicare beneficiaries who qualify for both Medicare and Medicaid account for 17 percent of the Medicare population and 19 percent of the Medicaid population (Gluck and Hanson, 2001; Health Care Financing Administration, 2000). These "dual eligibles" account for a total of 28 percent of Medicare expenditures and 35 percent of Medicaid expenditures. Native Americans eligible to receive services through IHS may also qualify for Medicaid if they satisfy income and other eligibility requirements, and those aged 65 and older may qualify for Medicare. Nearly 45 percent of veterans are 65 years and older and also qualify for Medicare (Van Diepen, 2001b). In addition, many Americans eligible for these programs have private supplemental insurance as well. Thus, patients and clinicians would surely benefit from greater consistency in quality enhancement requirements, measures, and processes across public and private insurance programs.

Table 2-1 provides a capsule summary of the six government health care programs. A more detailed description of the programs is provided in the following section. The broad trends affecting the needs and expectations of the programs' beneficiaries are then reviewed. The final section examines some key features of the programs beyond their quality enhancement processes.

MEDICARE[1]

Medicare provides health insurance to all individuals eligible for social security who are aged 65 and over, those eligible for social security because of a disability, and those suffering from end-stage renal disease (ESRD)—a total of about 40 million beneficiaries and growing. While

---

[1]Unless otherwise indicated, data in this section are based on Centers for Medicare and Medicaid Services, 1998, 2000c.

TABLE 2-1 Government Health Care Programs and Populations at a Glance

Characteristic	Medicare	Medicaid
Beneficiaries (2001)[a]	40 million	42.3 million
Eligibility	Eligibility for social security, (age 65 and over, end-stage-renal disease, or disabled)	Percent of federal poverty level and eligibility category (e.g., children, pregnant women, disabled)
Benefits	Basic acute care coverage, some preventive; high cost sharing, no prescription drugs	Comprehensive for both acute and chronic care plus institutional long-term care for the elderly, disabled, and mentally retarded; nominal cost sharing
Structure	Federal	Federal/state
Leading diagnoses	Hypertension, osteoporosis, chronic obstructive pulmonary disease, asthma, diabetes, heart disease, and stroke	Childbirth, asthma, hypertension, diabetes, congenital neurological and developmental disorders, mental health and substance abuse, tuberculosis, sexually transmitted diseases, and HIV/AIDS
Expenditures (2001)	$242.4 billion	$227.9 billion

[a]Some individuals are eligible for more than one government program.
SOURCES: Centers for Medicare and Medicaid Services, 1998, 2000a, 2000c, 2002a; Depart-

Medicare is 100 percent federally financed and operated, health care services are delivered almost entirely through the private sector. In 2002, about 87 percent of Medicare beneficiaries were covered by the Medicare fee-for-service (FFS) program; 13 percent of beneficiaries were enrolled in Medicare+Choice and cost-based health maintenance organizations (HMOs) (Centers for Medicare and Medicaid Services, 2002b). The Medicare population carries a heavy burden of chronic illness (never resolved conditions with continuing impairments that reduce the functioning of individuals)—78 percent of Medicare beneficiaries have at least one

SCHIP	VHA	DOD TRICARE	IHS
4.6 million	4 million	8.4 million	1.4 million
Generally up to 200% of federal poverty level and under age 19	Veterans with priority based on service discharge status and income	Active-duty military, their dependents, retirees	American Indians and Alaska Natives who belong to federally recognized tribes
Medicaid or actuarial equivalent of largest managed care plan in state; some cost sharing	Comprehensive chronic and acute care, including long-term institutional care; minimal cost sharing	Acute care coverage; no cost sharing for active duty personnel in military treatment facilities; some cost sharing for purchased care in civilian sector	Acute care, public health services, dental services, nutrition, community health, and other services
Federal/state	Federal	Federal	Federal/tribal
Not Available	Psychosis, substance abuse, heart failure, chronic obstructive pulmonary disease, pneumonia, chest pain, neuroses, arteriosclerosis, and digestive disorders	Childbirth, orthopedic injuries, chest pain, pneumonia, congestive heart failure, asthma, and depression	Diabetes, unintentional injuries, alcoholism, and substance abuse
$4.6 billion	$20.9 billion	$14.2 billion	$2.6 billion

ment of Health and Human Services, 1997, 2002; Indian Health Service, 2002; Medical Expenditure Panel Survey, 1998; TRICARE, 2002; Veterans Administration, 2001b.

chronic condition and 63 percent have two or more (Anderson, 2002). The over 30 percent of the Medicare population that has a physical and/or cognitive impairment accounts for about 60 percent of expenditures (see Figure 2-1). Medicare beneficiaries with three or more chronic conditions account for the bulk of program expenditures (see Figure 2-2). The most prevalent diagnoses in persons aged 65 and over—high blood pressure, osteoporosis, chronic obstructive pulmonary disease, asthma, diabetes, heart disease, and stroke—are all chronic illnesses requiring medical management over extended time periods and multiple settings (Medical Ex-

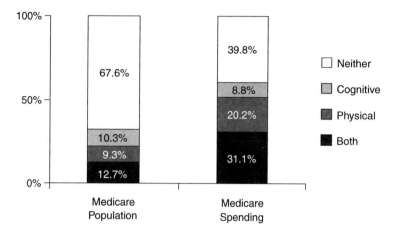

FIGURE 2-1 Medicare beneficiaries with cognitive and/or physical limitations as a percentage of beneficiary population and total Medicare expenditures, 1997. NOTE: A person with cognitive impairment has difficulty using the telephone or paying bills, or has Alzheimer's disease, mental retardation, or various other mental disorders. A person with physical impairment is someone reporting difficulty performing three or more activities of daily living.
SOURCE: Reprinted with permission from Moon and Storeygard, 2001.

penditure Panel Survey, 1998). The fastest-growing sectors in Medicare in terms of spending (though not the largest proportion of total program spending) have been home health, skilled nursing facilities, and hospice care, reflecting a shift in demand toward more chronic care.

MEDICAID[2]

Medicaid serves about 42 million people who are poor and who require health care services to achieve healthy growth and development goals or meet special health care needs. The program covers low-income people who meet its eligibility criteria, such as children, pregnant women, certain low-income parents, disabled adults, federal Supplemental Security Income (SSI) recipients (low-income children and adults with severe disability), and the medically needy (non-poor individuals with extraordinary medical expenditures who meet spend-down requirements generally for long-term care). There is a good deal of variability across states in the maximum income for eligibility.

---

[2]Unless otherwise indicated, data in this section are based on Centers for Medicare and Medicaid Services, 2000a.

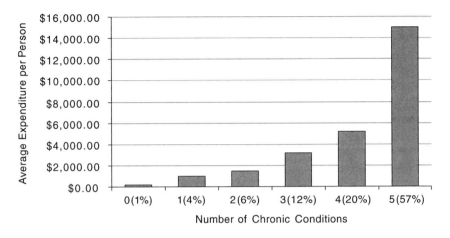

FIGURE 2-2 Medicare beneficiaries with five or more chronic conditions account for two-thirds of Medicare spending.
SOURCE: Centers for Medicare and Medicaid Services, 1999.

Medicaid is administered and financed jointly by the federal government and the states, although the federal government pays for over 50 percent of aggregate program expenditures (U.S. Government Printing Office, 2002). There is a good deal of variability in methods of health care delivery and financing across states. Medicaid programs rely extensively on private-sector health care providers, managed care plans, and community health centers to deliver services and, to a lesser degree, state, county, or other publicly owned facilities or programs. Nationwide, over half of the total Medicaid population is enrolled in Medicaid managed care arrangements. Institutionalized, disabled, dually eligible, and elderly beneficiaries are most likely to receive services through FFS payment arrangements.

The majority of Medicaid beneficiaries are children (54 percent), most under the age of 6 (see Figure 2-3). Each year, over one-third of all births in the United States are covered by Medicaid. While a minority of the program in terms of population (26 percent), the aged/blind/disabled account for 71 percent of program expenditures. Over half of Medicaid expenditures are for long-term care services, with the majority going to institutional long-term care providers (Centers for Medicare and Medicaid Services, 2000a).

While coordinated collection of Medicaid data from the states is lacking, other data sources indicate a substantial prevalence of chronic condi-

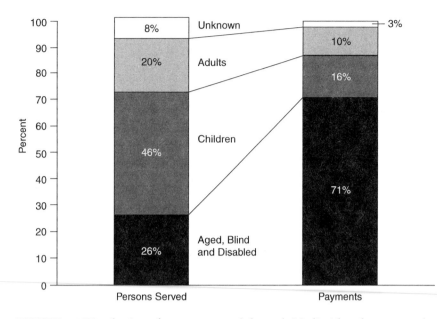

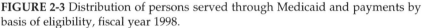

FIGURE 2-3 Distribution of persons served through Medicaid and payments by basis of eligibility, fiscal year 1998.
NOTE: Disabled children are included in the aged, blind and disabled category.
SOURCE: Centers for Medicare and Medicaid Services, 2000a.

tions in the program. These conditions include asthma, diabetes, neurological disorders, high blood pressure, mental illness, substance abuse, and HIV/AIDS (Centers for Medicare and Medicaid Services, 2001c; Medical Expenditure Panel Survey, 1996; Westmoreland, 1999).

STATE CHILDREN'S HEALTH INSURANCE PROGRAM[3]

Designed as a joint federal-state program, SCHIP was created in 1997 to provide health insurance to poor and near-poor children through age 18 without another source of insurance. Approximately 4.6 million children were enrolled in SCHIP as of fiscal year 2001 (Centers for Medicare and Medicaid Services, 2000b). SCHIP is targeted to children with incomes that exceed Medicaid eligibility requirements but remain under 200 percent of the federal poverty level (FPL) (Rosenbach et al., 2001). Some states

---

[3]Unless otherwise indicated, data in this section are based on Department of Health and Human Services, 1997.

have expanded SCHIP to children with family incomes up to 300 percent of FPL (Rosenbaum and Smith, 2001).

SCHIP operates as a block grant program to the states. States have the option of creating SCHIP programs as Medicaid expansions, as separate programs, or as combined programs (i.e., Medicaid expansions for some income levels and separate programs for higher income levels).

The SCHIP program has been implemented slowly and variably across states. Most states rely on managed care arrangements as their primary mechanism of service delivery for both healthy children and those with special health care needs.

VETERANS HEALTH ADMINISTRATION

VHA was established in 1946 as a separate division within the Veterans Administration to meet the health care needs of U.S. veterans (Veterans Administration, 2001b).[4] Veterans make up 10 percent of the nation's population, but only a minority receive care through VHA (Kizer, 1999; Van Diepen, 2001a). Eligibility is triaged according to the available budget; those with compensable, service-connected disabilities are assigned the highest priority (Veterans Administration, 2001a). VHA serves as a payer of last resort for treatment not related to service-connected disabilities that is provided through VHA facilities.

Health care is delivered through 22 regional health care systems, referred to as Veterans Integrated Service Networks (VISNs). Each VISN contains 7 to 10 hospitals, 25 to 30 ambulatory care clinics, 4 to 7 nursing homes, and other care delivery units (Kizer, 1999). Most clinical and administrative staff are employees of VHA.

Generally, the VHA population is older, low-income, and characterized by high rates of chronic illness (see Table 2-1). Approximately 19 percent of the total VHA population sought inpatient and outpatient mental health services (including those related to substance abuse) in 2000 (Van Diepen, 2001a).

DOD TRICARE[5]

DOD TRICARE encompasses two health care programs operated by the Department of Defense. TRICARE provides services to active-duty military personnel, their dependents, retirees under the age of 65 and their

---

[4]The VHA was initially established as the Department of Medicine and Surgery; it was succeeded in 1989 by the Veterans Health Services and Research Administration, and renamed the Veterans Health Administration in 1991.

[5]Unless otherwise indicated, data in this section are based on TRICARE, 2002.

spouses, and survivors. TRICARE for Life, a recent addition to the military health program, provides supplemental coverage (e.g., for prescription drugs) to the population aged 65 and over who enroll in Medicare Part B.

TRICARE is administered by the Office of the Assistant Secretary of Defense (Health Affairs). At the core of the program is a direct care system of military treatment facilities (MTFs), which provide most of the care delivered to active-duty personnel and over half of that provided to TRICARE beneficiaries overall. There is an MTF located at most major military facilities in the United States and abroad, each operated by one of the military services. TRICARE also has regional contracts with private-sector health plans to provide active-duty personnel with certain services not available through MTFs and to serve other beneficiaries. Non–active-duty beneficiaries may choose from among three program options: (1) TRICARE Prime, the lowest-cost plan, which assigns beneficiaries to a primary case manager, emphasizes preventive care, and makes use of MTFs whenever possible for specialty care; (2) TRICARE Extra, a preferred provider–type FFS discounted cost option; and (3) TRICARE Standard, the highest-cost plan, which provides maximal flexibility in selection of providers.

TRICARE is intended to ensure "force health protection." Active-duty personnel must be maintained at a level of health consistent with military demands according to a concept called "military readiness." The TRICARE program must also be capable of providing urgent and emergency care to injured soldiers, sometimes stationed in remote areas. Lastly, since the Gulf War, a great deal of attention has been focused on early detection of risks associated with the activities and settings of deployment (e.g., exposure to biological, chemical, and nuclear hazards and combat stress) and the ongoing monitoring of health consequences and effects of treatment (Institute of Medicine, 2000).

The TRICARE beneficiary population tends to be young and healthy. In addition to force health protection, the service needs of other TRICARE beneficiaries, mostly active-duty dependents, are sometimes described as basically babies and bones (Jennings, 2001). With the implementation of TRICARE for Life, TRICARE's elderly population can be expected to present health care needs similar to those of the Medicare population.

INDIAN HEALTH SERVICE[6]

IHS, an agency within the Department of Health and Human Services, is responsible for providing health services to members of federally

---

[6]The discussion in this section is based on data provided by Indian Health Service, 2002.

recognized American Indian and Alaska Native tribes. IHS currently provides health services to approximately 1.4 million American Indians and Alaska Natives belonging to more than 557 federally recognized tribes in 35 states.

The provision of these health services is based on treaties, judicial determinations, and acts of Congress that result in a unique government-to-government relationship between the tribes and the federal government. IHS, the principal health care provider, is organized as 12 area offices located throughout the United States. These 12 areas contain 550 health care delivery facilities operated by IHS and tribes, including: 49 hospitals; 214 health centers; and 280 health stations, satellite clinics, and Alaska village clinics. Almost 44 percent of the $2.6 billion IHS budget is transferred to the tribes to manage their own health care programs.

Poverty and low education levels strongly affect the health status of the Indian people. Approximately 26 percent of American Indians and Alaska Natives live below the poverty level, and more than one-third of Indians over age 25 who reside in reservation areas have not graduated from high school. Common inpatient diagnoses include diabetes, unintentional injuries, alcoholism, and substance abuse.

BROAD TRENDS AFFECTING THE NEEDS AND EXPECTATIONS OF BENEFICIARIES

In identifying ways to improve the quality enhancement processes of government health care programs, it is important to understand both the needs and expectations of today's beneficiaries and the trends likely to affect these needs and expectations in the future. As beneficiaries' needs and expectations evolve over time, so, too, must the government health care programs. This section highlights two important trends: the increase in chronic care needs and expectations for patient-centered care.

Chronic Care Needs

Trends in the epidemiology of health and disease and in medical science and technology have profound implications for health care delivery. Chronic conditions (defined as never resolved conditions, with continuing impairments that reduce the functioning of individuals) are now the leading cause of illness, disability, and death in the United States and affect almost half the U.S. population (Hoffman et al., 1996). Most older people have at least one chronic condition, and many have more than one (Administration on Aging, 2001). Fully 30 percent of those aged 65–74, and over 50 percent of those aged 75 and older report a limitation caused by a chronic condition (Administration on Aging, 2001). The proportion of children and adolescents with limitation of activity due to a chronic health condition more than tripled from 2 percent in 1960 to over 7 percent in the late 1990s (Newacheck and Halfon, 1998).

Thus, the majority of U.S. health care resources is now devoted to the treatment of chronic disease (Anderson and Knickman, 2001). This trend is strongly reflected in the government health care programs. In the Medicare and VHA programs, most of the beneficiaries have multiple chronic conditions. Diseases such as asthma, diabetes, hypertension, cancer, congestive heart failure, and mental health and cognitive disorders are important clinical concerns for all or nearly all of the programs.

The increasing prevalence of chronic illness challenges systems of care designed for episodic contact on an acute basis (Wagner et al., 1996). Hospitals and ambulatory settings are generally designed to provide acute care services, with limited communication among providers, and communication between providers and patients is often limited to periodic visits or hospitalizations for acute episodes. Serious chronic conditions, however, require ongoing and active medical management, with emphasis on secondary and tertiary prevention. The same patient may receive care in multiple settings, so that there is frequently a need to coordinate services across a variety of venues, including home, outpatient office or clinic setting, hospital, skilled nursing facility, and when appropriate, hospice.

There is mounting evidence that care for chronic conditions is seriously deficient. Fewer than half of U.S. patients with hypertension, depression, diabetes, and asthma are receiving appropriate preventive, acute, and chronic disease management services (Clark, 2000; Joint National Committee on Prevention, 1997; Legorreta et al., 2000; Wagner et al., 2001; Young et al., 2001). Health care is typically delivered by a mix of providers having separate, unrelated management systems, information systems, payment structures, financial incentives, and quality oversight for each segment of care, with disincentives for proactive, continuous care interventions (Bringewatt, 2001). For individuals with multiple chronic conditions, coordination of care and communication among providers are major problems that require immediate attention.

There are many efforts under way to develop new models of care capable of meeting the needs of the chronically ill. For example, Healthy Future Partnership for Quality, an initiative in Maine now in its fifth year, enrolls insured individuals (from leading health plans and the state Medicaid program) and uninsured individuals (covered by a 10 percent surcharge on the fee for each insured participant and paid by insurance companies) with chronic illness in an intensive care management program that provides patient education, improved access to primary care and preventive services, and disease management (Healthy Futures Partnership for Quality Project, 2002). The diabetes telemedicine collaborative in New York State (IDEATel, 2002) is a randomized controlled trial supported by CMS and others. It involves 1,500 patients, half of whom participate in home monitoring (using devices that read blood sugar, take pictures of skin and feet, and check blood pressure), intensive education on diabetes, and reminders and instructions on how to manage their disease.

The changing clinical needs of patients have important implications for government quality enhancement processes. These processes and the health care providers they monitor should be capable of assessing how well patients with chronic conditions are being managed across settings and time. This capability necessitates consolidation of all clinical and service use information for a patient across providers and sites, a most challenging task in a health care system that is highly decentralized and relies largely on paper medical records.

Patient-Centered Care

Patient-centered care is respectful of and responsive to individual patient preferences, needs, and values and ensures that patient values and circumstances guide all clinical decisions (Institute of Medicine, 2001). Informed patients participating actively in decisions about their own care appear to have better outcomes, lower costs, and higher functional status than those who take more passive roles (Gifford et al., 1998; Lorig et al., 1993, 1999; Stewert, 1995; Superio-Cabuslay et al., 1996; Van Korff et al., 1998). Most patients want to be involved in treatment decisions and to know about available alternatives (Guadagnoli and Ward, 1998); (Deber et al., 1996; Degner and Russell, 1988; Mazur and Hickam, 1997). Yet many physicians underestimate the extent to which patients want information about their care (Strull et al., 1984), and patients rarely receive adequate information for informed decision making (Braddock et al., 1999).

Patient-centered care is not a new concept, rather one that has been shaping the clinician and patient relationship for several decades. Authoritarian models of care have gradually been replaced by approaches that encourage greater patient access to information and input into decision making (Emanuel and Emanuel, 1992), though only to the extent that the patient desires such a role. Some patients may choose to delegate decision making to clinicians, while patients with cognitive impairments may not be capable of participating in decision making and may be without a close family member to serve as a proxy. Patients may also confront serious constraints in terms of covered benefits, copayments, and ability to pay (discussed below under benefits and copayments)

The recently released physician charter by the American Board of Internal Medicine (ABIM) Foundation, the American College of Physicians-

American Society of Internal Medicine (ACP-ASIM) Foundation, and the European Federation of Internal Medicine embodies three fundamental principles to guide the medical profession, including:

> *Principle of Patient Autonomy.* Physicians must have respect for patient autonomy. Physicians must be honest with their patients and empower them to make informed decisions about their treatment. Patients' decisions about their care must be paramount, as long as those decisions are in keeping with ethical practice and do not lead to demand for inappropriate care (American Board of Internal Medicine et al., 2002, p. 244).

The current focus on making the health care system more patient-centered stems at least in part from the growth in chronic care needs discussed above. Effective care of a person with a chronic condition is a collaborative process, involving extensive communication between the patient and the multidisciplinary team (Wagner et al., 2001). Patients and their families or other lay caregivers deliver much if not most of the care. Patients must have the confidence and skills to manage their condition, and they must understand their care plan (e.g., drug regimens and test schedules) to ensure proper and safe implementation. For many chronic diseases, such as asthma, diabetes, obesity, heart disease, and arthritis, effective ongoing management involves changes in diet, increased exercise, stress reduction, smoking cessation, and other aspects of lifestyle (Fox and Gruman, 1999; Lorig et al., 1999; Von Korff et al., 1997).

Pressures to make the care system more respectful of and responsive to the needs, preferences, and values of individual patients also stem from the increasing ethnic and cultural diversity that characterizes much of the United States. Although minority populations constitute less than 30 percent of the national population, in some states, such as California, they already constitute about 50 percent of the population (Institute for the Future, 2000). A culturally diverse population poses challenges that go beyond simple language competency and include the need to understand the effects of lifestyle and cultural differences on health status and health-related behaviors; the need to adapt treatment plans and modes of delivery to different lifestyles and familial patterns; the implications of a diverse genetic endowment among the population; and the prominence of nontraditional providers as well as family caregivers.

Although there has been a virtual explosion in Web-based health and health care information that might help patients and clinicians make more informed decisions, the information provided is of highly variable quality (Berland et al., 2001; Biermann et al., 1999; Landro, 2001). Some sites provide valid and reliable information. These include the National Library of Medicine's Medline Plus sites (Lindberg and Humphreys, 1999); the National Diabetes Education Program, launched by the Centers for Disease Control and Prevention and the National Institutes of Health (U.S. Government Printing Office, 2001); and the National Health Council's public education campaign. There are also notable efforts to provide consumers with comparative quality information on providers and health plans. Examples are the health plan report cards produced by the National Committee for Quality Assurance and by the Consumers Union/California HealthCare Foundation Partnership and nursing home quality reports produced by CMS (Centers for Medicare and Medicaid Services, 2001a; Consumers Union/California Healthcare Foundation Partnership, 2002; National Committee for Quality Assurance, 2002). These efforts are discussed further in Chapter 5. There is little doubt, however, that we are embarking on a long journey to determine how best to make valid and reliable information available to diverse audiences with different cultural and linguistic capabilities (Foote and Etheredge, 2002).

In general, communication with consumers is enhanced through the use of common terminology, standardized performance measures, and reporting formats that follow common conventions. At the program level, the predilection of each government program to design and operate its health care quality enhancement processes independently is a serious problem.

KEY PROGRAM FEATURES

Although the focus of this report is on quality enhancement processes, the committee believes it important to acknowledge other important program features—such as benefits, payment approaches, and program design and administration—that influence quality. Just as the quality enhancement processes of the government programs are being assessed in this report, these other aspects of program design must be evaluated in the future for alignment with the objectives of those processes.

Benefits and Copayments

Health insurance was established in the United States in the 1930s and 1940s as a way to help the average person cope with the high costs of hospital care (Stevens, 1989). Today hospital care, although still very expensive, consumes about one-third of the health care dollar, and other facets of health care, such as prescription medications (9 percent with a growth rate of 13.8 percent) have grown in importance (Centers for Medicare and Medicaid Services, 2002c; Strunk et al., 2002). Increased demand for these other facets of care reflects the growth in chronic care needs discussed earlier as well as new treatment options stemming from the extraordinary advances made in medical knowledge and technology, including minimally invasive surgery.

TABLE 2-2 Insurance Plans Covering Benefits Important to Chronically Ill Persons, 2000

Benefits[a]	% of Fortune 100[b]	Medicare	Medicaid Florida[c]
Prescription drugs	100	no	yes
Mental health outpatient services	100	yes	yes
Mental health inpatient services	100	yes	yes
Home health care	100	yes	yes
Physical therapy	100	yes	yes
Durable medical equipment	100	yes	yes
Occupational therapy	99	yes	yes
Speech therapy	99	yes	yes
Skilled nursing facilities	99	yes	yes
Chiropractor	97	yes	yes
Family counseling	50	yes	yes*
Dietitian–nutritionist	45	yes	yes*
Medical social worker	37	yes	yes*
Respite care	0	yes	yes
Personal care	0	no	yes*
Non-emergency transportation	0	no	yes
Home (environmental) modifications	0	no	yes*

*These services are provided to a limited subset of the state's Medicaid population.

[a]List of important benefits identified through focus group discussions and interviews with experts (Montenegro-Torres et al., 2001).

[b]Percentage of leading Fortune 100 companies providing this benefit to their employees in 2000 (Montenegro-Torres et al., 2001).

The benefit package of an insurance program has a direct effect on the likelihood of patients receiving needed health care services (Federman et al., 2001). Although there are frequent changes in the benefit packages of the various government health care programs, these modifications have not always kept pace with the needs, especially the chronic care needs, of the populations being served (Bringewatt, 2001).

When one assesses the extent to which the government health care programs provide coverage for benefits important to persons with chronic conditions, the results are mixed (see Table 2-2). The basic Medicare package, for example, generally does not cover outpatient prescription drugs or personal care, and coverage is very limited for preventive services, nursing home services, family counseling, and dietitian–nutritionist services. Medicare payment mechanisms are designed for acute care, often by a single provider; there is no Medicare payment mechanism that recognizes care delivered by a team of providers to an individual with mul-

Medicaid Arizona[c]	Medicaid Connecticut[c]	VHA	TRICARE
yes	yes	yes	yes
yes	yes	yes	yes
yes	yes	yes	yes
yes	yes	yes	yes
yes	yes	yes	yes
yes	yes	yes	yes
yes	yes	yes	yes
yes	yes	yes	yes
yes	yes	yes	yes
no	yes	yes	no
yes	yes	yes	yes
yes	yes	yes	outpatient
no	yes*	yes	yes
yes	yes	yes	some cases under hospice
yes	no	yes	no
yes	yes	yes	no
yes	yes*	yes	no

[c]There is a good deal of variability across states in covered benefits. These three states were selected at random, and may or may not be representative of Medicaid plans in general.

SOURCES: Agency for Health Care Administration, 2002; Anderson, 2002; Arizona Health Care Cost Containment System, 2002; Centers for Medicare and Medicaid Services, 2001b; and Connecticut Department of Social Services, 2002.

tiple chronic conditions or that rewards prevention efforts such as extensive patient education for self-care.

Other government programs offer important benefits in specific areas. VHA provides extensive mental health outpatient and inpatient services, especially for veterans with service-related disabilities. Medicaid provides residential care to the disabled and mentally retarded and long-term care for the elderly as a major part of program spending. Its benefit package is very comprehensive, including complex therapies for chronic conditions and congenital neurological disorders, such as cerebral palsy and Down syndrome, although states vary substantially in the scope of such benefits. Both Medicaid and SCHIP programs cover outpatient prescription medications. Note that IHS is not included in Table 2-2 because it is not an entitlement program or an insurance plan; therefore, it has no established benefit package (Indian Health Service, 2001). It is estimated that funds appropriated to IHS by Congress cover approximately 60 percent of the health care needs of beneficiaries (Indian Health Service, 2001)

Cost-sharing provisions are also important. Persons with chronic conditions are the heaviest users of health care services. Deductibles and especially copayments can be sizable for these individuals. Some government health care programs, such as VHA, have minimal cost-sharing provisions, while others, especially Medicare, make more extensive use of such provisions.

Also important is how the different programs interpret "medical necessity." Even when a service is covered, payment for that service to a particular patient can be denied because of failure to meet a medical necessity criterion. In some instances, the quantity and duration of certain repetitive services may be limited unless the person shows functional improvement, not just stability or a slowing of decline (Anderson et al., 1998).

The committee believes that each of the six government health care programs should review its benefit package and medical necessity criteria to identify enhancements in coverage or cost sharing that would facilitate the provision of more appropriate care to today's beneficiaries. Such analyses should be conducted under alternative financial scenarios, including budget neutrality and varying levels of growth in expenditures. Efforts should also be made to understand how well the benefit packages of various government health care programs meet the needs of vulnerable populations and how well these packages fit together for those who are dual- or triple-eligible.

Payment Approaches

Efforts to improve quality of care will be far more effective if implemented in an environment that encourages and rewards excellence. Unfortunately, current methods of payment to health plans and providers have the unintended consequence of working against quality objectives. This is true for both capitated and FFS payment methods.

Capitation is a payment arrangement in which health plans are paid a fixed amount for each enrollee under their care, regardless of the level of services needed by and actually provided to the person. Some health plans also pay physicians on a capitated basis for certain outpatient care, putting them at some degree of financial risk.

Capitated payment rates are usually based on the average cost per enrollee of the enrolled group, often with adjustments for demographic characteristics (e.g., age and sex). Capitation rates are usually not adjusted for the health status of the enrolled population. Therefore, health plans and providers receive the same payment for someone who is less healthy and more likely to use a large number of services, such as a person with a chronic condition, as they do for someone who is healthier and likely to use no or fewer services during the year.

Health plans or clinicians that develop exemplary care programs for persons with chronic conditions may, as a result, attract a disproportionate share of these individuals. Under capitated payment systems, this situation has a highly negative financial impact on the health plan and providers (Luft, 1995; Maguire et al., 1998). Persons with chronic conditions are more likely both to use services and to use a greater number of services during the year than those without chronic conditions. In 1996, for example, mean health care expenditures for a person with one or more chronic conditions were nearly 4 times the overall average ($3,546 versus $821) (Partnerships for Solutions, forthcoming). The average number of inpatient days per year is 0.2 for persons with no chronic conditions compared to 4.6 for those with five or more such conditions.

Risk adjustment is a mechanism designed to ensure that payments to health plans and other capitated providers more accurately reflect the expected cost of providing health care services to the population enrolled. Capitated plans and providers caring for a population that includes less healthy, higher-cost enrollees should receive higher payments. As more states require their entire Medicaid populations, including those who are disabled and have high health care needs, to enroll in managed care, adjustment of payments becomes even more necessary to ensure quality of care for enrollees (Maguire et al., 1998). Some states have addressed this issue. Michigan, for example, has created a separately funded capitated option for children with special health care needs (Department of Health and Human Services, 2000).

Numerous options exist for risk-adjusting payments, but their application in government health care programs has been limited (Ellis et al., 1996; Hornbrook and Goodman, 1996; Newhouse et al., 1997; Starfield et al., 1991). The Medicare+Choice program has initiated demonstration projects to pilot the application of capitated payments adjusted for health status (Centers for Medicare and Medicaid Services, 2000d).

Regardless of whether the beneficiary is enrolled in an indemnity or capitated plan, the physicians on the front line of care delivery in the private sector are generally compensated under FFS payment methods (Center for Studying Health System Change, 2001; Institute of Medicine, 2001). FFS is the most common method of payment to physicians under Medicare, Medicaid, and SCHIP.

Under FFS payment, physicians have strong financial incentives to increase their volume of billable services (e.g., visits and office-based procedures and tests). Sometimes the incentives of FFS or other physician payment methods are attenuated by incentives (e.g., bonuses) tied to performance (e.g., measures of safety, clinical quality, service), but this is not the norm. In a 1998–1999 survey of a nationally representative sample of physicians, fewer than 30 percent indicated that their compensation was affected by performance-based incentives, a result similar to findings from a survey conducted in 1996–1997 (Stoddard et al., 2002). When they are used, performance-based incentives are more likely to be tied to patient satisfaction (24 percent) and quality measures (19 percent) than to measures that may restrain care, such as profiling (14 percent).

The principal "reimbursable event" under FFS is a face-to-face encounter between a physician and patient, which may or may not trigger other reimbursable events, such as diagnostic tests and minor office procedures. Services such as e-mail communications, telephone consultations, patient education classes, and care coordination are important for the ongoing management of chronic conditions, but they are not reimbursable events. Moreover, physicians who communicate with patients through e-mail or telephone to emphasize patient education, self-management of chronic conditions, and to coordinate care may experience a reduction in overall revenues if these uncompensated services have the effect of reducing patient demand for or time available to devote to reimbursable face-to-face encounters.

There is no perfect payment method; all methods have advantages and disadvantages. FFS contributes to overuse of billable services (e.g., face-to-face encounters, ancillary tests, procedures) and underuse of preventive services, counseling, medications, and other services often not covered under indemnity insurance programs. Overuse, especially the provision of services that expose patients to more potential harm than good, is a serious quality-of-care and cost concern. On the other hand, capitated payments may contribute to underuse—the failure to provide services from which patients would likely benefit. This is especially true when there is a good deal of turnover among plan enrollees so that the long-term cost consequences of underuse tend to be borne by another insurer. Although particular payment methods may contain a bias towards underuse or overuse, it is important to note that the quality-of-care literature contains ample evidence of both phenomena occurring in both FFS and capitated payment systems, reinforcing the notion that payment is but one, albeit an important, factor influencing care (Chassin and Galvin, 1998).

The committee believes enhancements can be made in both capitated and FFS payment approaches to encourage the provision of quality health care. It should also be noted that there are some promising efforts under way to design alternative payment approaches and evaluate their impact on quality. The National Health Care Purchasing Institute, a nonprofit research institute supported by The Robert Wood Johnson Foundation, has identified various incentive models that might be effective in motivat-

---

BOX 2-1
Possible Financial Incentive Models for Rewarding Providers for Quality Improvements

Quality bonuses—An additional annual payment is made to a provider (usually 5 to 10 percent of annual compensation) based on the achievement of certain performance goals.

Compensation at risk—A portion of a provider's compensation is placed "at risk" based on the provider's performance on quality measures.

Performance fee schedule—A provider's fee schedule is linked to performance on a set of quality measures (e.g., providers achieving exemplary levels of performance might receive 115 percent of the base fee schedule, while poor performers might receive 85 percent).

Variable cost sharing for patients—A patient's deductible and copayments are linked to the provider's performance on a set of quality measures (e.g., patients who see providers with high performance scores have lower cost sharing than those who see the poorer performing providers).

SOURCE: Adapted from Bailit Health Purchasing, 2002b.

---

ing providers to improve their performance; some of these models are highlighted in Box 2-1. Numerous efforts are under way to test some of these approaches. Examples include the following:

• The Buyers Health Care Action Group, an employer coalition in Minnesota, provides gold ($100,000) and silver ($50,000) awards to care systems for performance on quality improvement projects (Bailit Health Purchasing, 2002a)

• PacifiCare in California has developed a quality index that profiles providers on the basis of measures of clinical quality, patient safety, service quality, and efficiency. This information is used to reward providers on the basis of their performance, as well as to construct a tiered system of premiums, copayments, and coinsurance rates for enrollees that vary inversely with provider performance in terms of quality and efficiency (Ho, 2002)

• The Employers' Coalition on Health in Rockford, Illinois, makes incentive payments to provider groups based on whether the group completes care flowsheets on 95 percent of its diabetic encounters and maintains hemoglobin A1c levels below 7.5 for the majority of patients. Incentive payments to medical groups have been approximately $28,000 per year ($3.60 per member per year) (Bailit Health Purchasing, 2002a)

• Blue Shield of California has introduced a variable cost-sharing model under which patients pay either an additional $200 copayment or 10 percent of the hospital's fee each time they are admitted to a hospital that is not on Blue Shield's preferred list. Blue Shield rates hospitals on the basis of measures of quality, safety, patient satisfaction, and efficiency (Freudenheim, 2002)

• General Motors' value-based purchasing approach rates health plans according to their performance on various clinical quality measures, patient satisfaction measures, NCQA accreditation results, and cost-effectiveness measures, and adjusts employee out-of-pocket contributions so that those choosing the best-ranked plans have the lowest contributions (Salber and Bradley, 2001).

It may be hoped that much more will be known about the impact of various financial and non-financial incentive models in the near future. The Robert Wood Johnson Foundation (National Health Care Purchasing Institute, 2002) has recently announced an initiative entitled "Rewarding Results," which will provide support for payment demonstrations that reward improvements in quality. This initiative is being evaluated under an Agency for Healthcare Research and Quality contract.

Program Design and Administration

Benefits coverage and payment methods are among the most important design features of the six government health care programs reviewed in this report, but they are not the only ones that influence the likelihood of patients receiving high-quality care. Other important features include delivery system and provider choices, fluctuations in eligibility and delivery system options, and administrative efficiency.

In some government health care programs, consumers have multiple options in terms of delivery system and choice of providers, while in others the options are more limited. Under Medicare, 87 percent of beneficiaries have chosen to enroll in FFS arrangements, which provide extensive choice of clinicians and hospitals. Most Medicare beneficiaries who live in metropolitan areas also have the option of enrolling in Medicare+Choice plans, enrollment that historically has been associated with enhanced benefits for little or no additional out-of-pocket expense. Enrollment in managed care is mandatory for the majority of the Medicaid population in most states, and in some instances, there is little or no choice of plan. DOD TRICARE, the VHA, and IHS programs are all structured to encourage, and in some cases require, use of their own health care delivery systems, which are similar to group or staff-model health plans.

Studies of the clinical quality (in terms of both medical care processes and patient outcomes) in managed care and indemnity settings consistently find little or no difference between the two (Chassin and Galvin, 1998; Miller and Luft, 1993; Schuster et al., 1998). But it is clear that some consumers have strong preferences for one delivery system over another, and that most prefer to have choice (Gawande et al., 1998; Ullman et al., 1997). Limited choice of health plans may or may not seriously constrain the choice of clinicians and hospitals, since plan networks vary greatly in size and structure (Lake and Gold, 1999). In the private sector, there has been a pronounced trend in recent years toward larger networks of providers in response to consumer demand for more extensive choice (Draper et al., 2002; Lesser and Ginsburg, 2000). In the absence of comparative quality information on providers, consumers apparently equate choice with quality.

The design and financing of some government health care programs result in frequent changes in eligibility and delivery system options that disrupt patterns of care delivery. Since the implementation of changes in Medicare payment policies stemming from enactment of the Balanced Budget Act of 1997, there has been a steady erosion of health plans participating in the Medicare+Choice program. Since 1998, 2.2 million Medicare beneficiaries have been involuntarily disenrolled from Medicare+Choice plans, affecting approximately 5 percent of beneficiaries in 2002. Of the health plans that remain, the proportion offering prescription drug coverage during the period 1999 through 2002 dropped from 73 to 66 percent, and the proportion charging zero premiums to beneficiaries from 62 to 39 percent (Gold and McCoy, 2002). Under Medicaid, beneficiaries move in and out of the program as their eligibility changes in accordance with minor fluctuations in income, causing beneficiaries to lose contact with providers and further complicating the tracking of care. For many eligible children and women, the re-enrollment process is initiated only when they present themselves at a hospital or physician's office seeking service for an illness; this process results in adverse selection in capitated plans.

Lastly, efforts must be made to reduce administrative burden. In recent years, there has been a steady growth in regulatory requirements in most if not all of the government health care programs. The Secretary's Advisory Committee on Regulatory Reform estimates that about two regulations are published each week, resulting in the promulgation of more than 120 regulations in each of the last two years (Wood, 2002). The American Hospital Association (2002) has identified 100 new or revised regulations pertaining to hospitals that have been issued by federal agencies since 1997, of which 57 are significant. Some of these regulations relate to quality enhancement processes and data requirements, while others relate to such areas as payment, patient confidentiality and privacy, and fraud and abuse.

Regulatory oversight is necessary, but it must be balanced and efficient. The current practice of promulgating separate regulations for each type of provider (e.g., hospital, home health agency, nursing home, ambulatory care provider) has produced excessive burdens and barriers to the provision of coordinated care. Unnecessary regulations frustrate clinicians and reduce the time available to devote to patient care. They can also interfere with the movement of individuals across settings, thus hampering the transition from hospital to nursing home to home health agency, for example.

Regulatory burden must also be fair. For example, the quality measurement and reporting requirements applied to Medicare+Choice plans should be applied to FFS Medicare institutional and individual providers. These issues are addressed further in Chapters 3 and 4.

In summary, while technically comprising separate areas of analysis, the issues of benefits, payment, program design, and administration are inextricably linked to achieving consistent levels of high-quality care.

REFERENCES

Administration on Aging. 2001. "Profile of Older Americans: 2000." Online. Available at http://www.aoa.dhhs.gov/aoa/STATS/profile/default.htm. [accessed Aug. 3, 2001].

Agency for Health Care Administration. 2002. "Florida Medicaid Program: Summary of Services." Online. Available at http://www.fdhc.state.fl.us/Medicaid/sos.pdf [accessed Apr. 8, 2002].

American Board of Internal Medicine, ACP-ASIM Foundation, and European Federation of Internal Medicine. 2002 . Medical professionalism in the new millennium: a physician charter. *Ann Intern Med* 136 (3).

American Hospital Association. 2002. *Patients or Paperwork? The Regulatory Burden Facing America's Hospitals.* Washington DC: PricewaterhouseCoopers for American Hospital Association.

Anderson, G. 2002. "Testimony Before the Subcommittee on Health of the House Committee on Ways and Means Hearing on Promoting Disease Management in Medicare." Online. Available at http://waysandmeans.house.gov/health/107cong/4-16-02/4-16ande.htm [accessed May 3, 2002].

Anderson, G., M. A. Hall, and T. R. Smith. 1998. When courts review medical appropriateness. *Med Care* 36 (8):1295-302.

Anderson, G., and J. R. Knickman. 2001. Changing the chronic care system to meet people's needs. *Health Aff* 20 (6):146-60.

Arizona Health Care Cost Containment System. 2002. "2001 AHCCCS Overview: Table of Contents." Online. Available at http://www.ahcccs.state.az.us/Publications/Overview/2001/contents.asp [accessed Apr. 8, 2002].

Bailit Health Purchasing. 2002a. *Ensuring Quality Health Plans: A Purchaser's Toolkit for Using Incentives.* Washington DC: National Health Care Purchasing Institute.

———. 2002b. *Provider Incentive Models for Improving Quality of Care.* Washington DC: National Health Care Purchasing Institute.

Berland, G. K., M. N. Elliott, L. S. Morales, J. I. Algazy, R. L. Kravitz, M. S. Broder, D. E. Kanouse, J. A. Munoz, J. A. Puyol, M. Lara, K. E. Watkins, H. Yang, and E. A. McGlynn. 2001. Health information on the Internet: accessibility, quality, and readability in English and Spanish. *JAMA* 285 (20):2612-21.

Biermann, S., G. Golladay, M. Greenfield, and L. Baker. 1999. Evaluation of Cancer Information on the Internet. *Cancer* 86 (3): 381-90.

Braddock III, C., K. Edwards, N. Hasenberg, T. Laidley, and W. Levinson. 1999. Informed decision making in outpatient practice: time to get back to basics. *JAMA* 282 (24):2313-20.

Bringewatt, R. 2001. Making a business case for high-quality chronic illness care. *Health Aff (Millwood)* 6 (20):59-60.

Center for Studying Health System Change. 2001. *Community Tracking Study Physician Survey 1998-1999 [United States]*. Washington DC: ICPSR.

Centers for Medicare and Medicaid Services. 1998. "A Profile of Medicare." Online. Available at http://www.hcfa.gov/pubforms/chartbk.pdf [accessed Aug. 22, 2001].

Centers for Medicare and Medicaid Services. 1999. *Medicare Standard Analytic File*. Washington DC: U.S. Department of Health and Human Services.

Centers for Medicare and Medicaid Services. 2000a. "A Profile of Medicaid: Chartbook 2000." Online. Available at http://www.hcfa.gov/stats/stats.htm [accessed Oct. 16, 2001a].

———. 2000b. "State Children's Health Insurance Program (SCHIP) Aggregate Enrollment Statistics for the 50 States and the District of Columbia for Federal Fiscal Year (FFY) 2000." Online. Available at http://www.hcfa.gov/init/fy2000.pdf [accessed Oct. 16, 2001b].

———. 2000c. "Medicare Profile Chart Book from the 35th Anniversary Event." Online. Available at http://www.hcfa.gov/stats/stats.htm [accessed Oct. 16, 2001c].

———. 2000d. "Operational Policy Letter #126 re: Reconciliation of Calendar Year (CY) 2000 Payments Based on Changes in Risk Adjuster Factors/Enhanced Monthly Membership Reporting." Online. Available at http://www.hcfa.gov/medicare/opl126.htm [accessed Apr. 10, 2002d].

———. 2001a. "Nursing Home Compare - Home." Online. Available at http://www.medicare.gov/NHCompare/home.asp [accessed May 6, 2002a].

———. 2001b. "Your Medicare Benefits." Online. Available at http://www.medicare.gov/Publications/Pubs/pdf/yourmb.pdf [accessed Apr. 8, 2002b].

———. 2001c. "Fact Sheet: Center for Medicaid and State Operations; Medicaid and Acquired Immunodeficiency Syndrome (AIDS) and Human Immunodeficiency Virus (HIV) Infection." Online. Available at http://www.hcfa.gov/medicaid/obs11.htm [accessed Aug. 15, 2001c].

———. 2002a. "State Children's Health Insurance Program: Fiscal year 2001 annual enrollment report." Online. Available at http://www.cms.hhs.gov/schip/schip01.pdf [accessed June 28, 2002a].

———. 2002b. "Program Information on Medicare, Medicaid, SCHIP, and other programs of the Centers for Medicare & Medicaid Services." Online. Available at http://cms.hhs.gov/charts/series/sec3-b1.pdf [accessed Aug. 14, 2002b].

———. 2002c. "Where the Nations's Health Dollar Came From and Where it Went." Online. Available at http://cms.hhs.gov/statistics/nhe/historical/chart.asp [accessed Sept. 26, 2002c].

Chassin, M., and R. Galvin. 1998. The urgent need to improve health care quality: Institute of Medicine National Roundtable on Quality. *JAMA* 280 (11):1000-05.

Clark, C. 2000. Promoting early diagnosis and treatment of type 2 diabetes. *Journal of the American Medical Association* 284 (3):363-65.

Connecticut Department of Social Services. 2002. "State of Connecticut Department of Social Services." Online. Available at http://www.dss.state.ct.us [accessed Apr. 8, 2002].

Consumers Union/California Healthcare Foundation Partnership. 2002. "Guide to California Medicare HMOs: All Medicare HMOs are NOT alike." Online. Available at http://admin.chcf.org/documents/hmoguide/GuideToCaliforniaMedicareHMOs.pdf [accessed May 6, 2002].

Deber, R., N. Kraetschmer, and J. Irvine. 1996. What role do patients wish to play in treatment decision making? *Arch Int Med* 156 (1414-20).

Degner, L., and C. Russell. 1988. Preferences for treatment control among adults with cancer. *Res Nurs Health* 11:367-74.

Department of Health and Human Services. 1997. "State Children's Health Insurance Program homepage." Online. Available at http://www.hcfa.gov/init/children.htm [accessed Apr. 5, 2002].

———. 2000. *Secretary of the Department of Health and Human Services, Report to Congress: Safeguards for Individuals with Special Health Care Needs Enrolled in Medicaid Managed Care.* Washington DC: U.S. Department of Health and Human Services.

———. 2002. *2002 CMS Statistics. CMS Publication No. 03437.* Baltimore MD: U.S. Department of Health and Human Services.

Draper, D. A., R. E. Hurley, C. S. Lesser, and B. C. Strunk. 2002. The changing face of managed care. *Health Aff (Millwood)* 21 (1):11-23.

Ellis, R., G. Pope, L. Iezzoni, et al. 1996. Diagnosis-based risk adjustment for Medicare capitation payments. *Health Care Financ Rev* 17 (3):101-28.

Emanuel, E., and L. Emanuel. 1992. Four models of the physician-patient relationship. *JAMA* 267 (16):2221-6.

Federman, A. D., A. S. Adams, D. Ross-Degnan, S. B. Soumerai, and J. Z. Ayanian. 2001. Supplemental insurance and use of effective cardiovascular drugs among elderly Medicare beneficiaries with coronary heart disease. *JAMA* 286 (14):1732-39.

Foote, S., and L. Etheredge. 2002. *Strategies to Improve Consumer Health Information Services. Health Insurance Reform Project.* Washington DC: The George Washington University.

Fox, D., and J. Gruman, Milbank Memorial Fund and Center for the Advancement of Health. 1999. "Patients as Effective Collaborators in Managing Chronic Conditions." Online. Available at http://www.milbank.org/990811chronic.html [accessed 2001].

Freudenheim, M. June 26, 2002. Quality goals in incentives for hospitals. *New York Times.* Sect. Late Edition: Final, Section C, Page 1, Column 5.

Gawande, A. A., R. Blendon, M. Brodie, J. M. Benson, L. Levitt, and L. Hugick. 1998. Does dissatisfaction with health plans stem from having no choices? *Health Aff (Millwood)* 17 (5):184-94.

Gifford, A. L., D. D. Laurent, V. M. Gonzales, M. A. Chesney, and K. R. Lorig. 1998. Pilot randomized trial of education to improve self-management skills of men with symptomatic HIV/AIDS. *J Acquir Immune Defic Syndr Hum Retrovirol* 18 (2):136-44.

Gluck, M., and K. W. Hanson. 2001. *Medicare Chart Book.* Menlo Park CA: Henry J. Kaiser Family Foundation.

Gold, M., and J. McCoy. 2002. Monitoring Medicare and choice: fast facts. Choice continues to erode in 2002. *Mathematica Policy Research* 7:1-2.

Guadagnoli, E., and P. Ward. 1998. Patient participation in decision-making. *Soc Sci Med* 47 (3):329-39.

Health Care Financing Administration. 2000. *A Profile of Medicaid: Chart Book.* Baltimore MD: U.S. Department of Health and Human Services.

Healthy Futures Partnership for Quality Project. 2002. Healthy Futures and the Maine Center for Public Health, unpublished paper.

Ho, S. (Pacificare). 13 May 2002. Provider quality index. Personal communication to Janet Corrigan.

Hoffman, C., D. Rice, and H. Sung. 1996. Persons with chronic conditions. Their prevalence and costs. *JAMA* 276 (18):1473-79.

Hornbrook, M., and M. Goodman. 1996. Chronic disease, functional health status, and demographics: a multi-dimensional approach to risk adjustment. *Health Serv Res* 31 (3):283-307.

IDEATel. 2002. "Informatics for Diabetes Education and Telemedicine." Online. Available at http://www.ideatel.org/info.html [accessed July 30, 2002].

Indian Health Service. 2001. "Indian Health Service: Customer Services." Online. Available at http://www.ihs.gov/GeneralWeb/HelpCenter/CustomerServices/approp.asp [accessed Aug. 14, 2002].

———. 2002. "Indian Health Service Homepage." Online. Available at http://www.ihs.gov [accessed Feb. 14, 2002].

Institute for the Future. 2000. *Health and Health Care, 2010: The Forecast, the Challenge. Based on 1998 data provided by the Department of Finance, State of California.* San Francisco CA: Institute for the Future.

Institute of Medicine. 2000. *Protecting Those Who Serve: Strategies to Protect the Health of Deployed U.S. Forces.* Washington DC: National Academy Press.

———. 2001. *Crossing the Quality Chasm: A New Health System for the 21st Century.* Washington DC: National Academy Press.

Jennings, B. (TMA). September 2001. TRICARE. Personal communication to Barbara Smith.

Joint National Committee on Prevention. 1997. Detection, evaluation, and treatment of high blood pressure, Sixth Report. *Arch Intern Med* 157 (21):2413-46.

Kizer, K. 1999. The new VA: a national laboratory for health care quality management. *Am J Med Qual* 14 (1):3-20.

Lake, T., and M. Gold. 1999. *Health plan selection and payment of health care providers.* Washington DC: MedPAC.

Landro, L. Nov. 12, 2001. Getting reliable health information. *Wall Street Journal.*

Legorreta, A. P., X. Zaher, C. A. Liu, and D. E. Jatulis. 2000. Variation in managing asthma: experience at the medical group level in California. *Am J Manag Care* 6 (4):445-53.

Lesser, C. S., and P. B. Ginsburg. 2000. Update on the nation's health care system: 1997-1999. *Health Aff (Millwood)* 19 (6):206-16.

Lindberg, D., and B. Humphreys. 1999. A time for change for medical informatics in the USA. *Yearbook of Medical Informatics* 53 (7).

Lorig, K., P. Mazonson, and H. Holman. 1993. Evidence suggesting that health education for self management in chronic arthritis has sustained health benefits while reducing health care costs. *Arthritis Rheumatism* 36 (4):439-46.

Lorig, K. R., D. S. Sobel, A. L. Stewart, B. W. Brown Jr, A. Bandura, P. Ritter, V. M. Gonzalez, D. D. Laurent, and H. R. Holman. 1999. Evidence Suggesting that a Chronic Disease Self-Management Program Can Improve Health Status While Reducing Hospitalization: A Randomized Trial. *Med Care* 37 (1):5-14.

Luft, H. 1995. Potential methods to reduce risk selection and its effects. *Inquiry* 32:23-32.

Maguire, A. M., N. R. Powe, B. Starfield, J. Andrews, J. P. Weiner, and G. F. Anderson. 1998. "Carving out" conditions from global capitation rates: protecting high-cost patients, physicians, and health plans in a managed care environment. *Am J Manag Care* 4 (6):797-806.

Mazur, D. J., and D. H. Hickam. 1997. Patients' preferences for risk disclosure and role in decision making for invasive medical procedures. *J Gen Intern Med* 12 (2):114-17.

Medical Expenditure Panel Survey. 1996. CCS clinical conditions from MEPS, 1996; for persons with primary medicaid coverage during year, all ages; estimated number of persons with medicaid coverage: sorted by total cost of chronic condition.

———. 1998. Counts and expenditures for specific conditions; MEPS 1998 data.

Miller, R., and H. Luft. 1993. Managed care: past evidence and potential trends. *Front Health Serv Manage* 9 (3):3-37.

Montenegro-Torres, B., T. Engelhardt, M. Thamer, and G. Anderson. 2001. Are Fortune 100 companies responsive to chronically ill workers? *Health Aff* 20 (4):209-19.

Moon, M., and M. Storeygard. 2001. *One-Third at Risk: The Special Circumstances of Medicare Beneficiaries with Health Problems.* New York NY: The Commonwealth Fund.

National Committee for Quality Assurance. 2002. "NCQA Report Cards." Online. Available at http://hprc.ncqa.org/menu.asp [accessed May 6, 2002].

National Health Care Purchasing Institute. 2002. "Rewarding Results." Online. Available at http://www.nhcpi.net/rewardingresults/index.cfm [accessed Apr. 22, 2002].

Newacheck, P. W., and N. Halfon. 1998. Prevalence and impact of disabling chronic conditions in childhood. *Am J Public Health* 88 (4):610-7.

Newhouse, J., M. Buntin, and J. Chapman. 1997. Risk adjustment and Medicare: taking a closer look. *Health Aff (Millwood)* 16 (5):26-43.

Partnerships for Solutions. forthcoming. *Medicare Expenditures Increase with the Number of Chronic Conditions; 1996 MEPS data.* Baltimore MD: John Hopkins University.

Rosenbach, M., M. Ellwood, J. Czajka, C. Irvin, W. Coupe, and B. Quinn. 2001. *Implementation of the State Children's Health Insurance Program: Momentum is Increasing After a Modest Start.* Princeton, NJ: Mathematica Policy Research, Inc.

Rosenbaum, S., and B. M. Smith. 2001. *Policy Brief #1: State SCHIP Design and The Right to Coverage.* Washington, D.C.: Center for Health Services Research and Policy, George Washington University School of Public Health.

Salber, P., and B. Bradley. 2001. "Perspective: Salber and Bradley Web Exclusive." Online. Available at http://www.healthaffairs.org/WebExclusives/Salber_Bradley_ Perspective_ Web_Excl_112801.htm [accessed Aug. 14, 2002].

Schuster, M. A., E. A. McGlynn, and R. H. Brook. 1998. How good is the quality of health care in the United States? *Milbank Q* 76 (4):517-63.

Starfield, B., J. Weiner, L. Mumford, and D. Steinwachs. 1991. Ambulatory care groups: a categorization of diagnoses for research and management. *Health Serv Res* 26 (1):53-74.

Stevens, R. 1989. *In Sickness and Wealth: American Hospitals in the 20th Century.* New York: Basic Books, Inc.

Stewert, M. 1995. Effective physician-patient communication and health outcomes: a review. *Can Med Assoc J* 152 (9):1423-33.

Stoddard, J., J. Grossman, and L. Rudell. 2002. *Physicians More Likely to Face Quality Incentives Than Incentives That May Restrain Care.* Washington DC: Center for Studying Health System Change.

Strull, W., B. Lo, and G. Charles. 1984. Do patients want to participate in medical decision-making? *JAMA* 252 (21):2990-2994.

Strunk, B., P. Ginsburg, and J. Gabel. 2002. "Data Bulletin No. 22: tracking health care cost. Hospital spending spurs double-digit increase in 2001." Online. Available at http://www.hschange.com/CONTENT/472/ [accessed Sept. 26, 2002].

Superio-Cabuslay, E., M. Ward, and K. Lorig. 1996. Patient education interventions in osteoarthritis and rheumatoid arthritis: a meta-analytic comparison with non-steroidal antiinflammatory drug treatment. *Arthritis Care Res* 9 (4):292-301.

TRICARE. 2002. "TRICARE Homepage." Online. Available at http://www.tricare.osd.mil/ [accessed Apr. 3, 2002].

U.S. Government Printing Office. 2001. *National Diabetes Education Program. "Changing the Way Diabetes is Treated."* Washington DC: U.S. Government Printing Office.

———. 2002. "Chapter 4 Promoting Health Care Quality and Access." *Economic Report of the President.*

Ullman, R., J. W. Hill, E. C. Scheye, and R. K. Spoeri. 1997. Satisfaction and choice: a view from the plans. *Health Aff (Millwood)* 16 (3):209-17.

Van Diepen, L. (VA). 19 July 2001a. VA Stats. Personal communication to Barbara Smith.

Van Diepen, L. (VA). 14 August 2001b. RE: # VA hospitals. Personal communication to Elaine Swift.

Van Korff, M., E. Moore, K. Lorig, D. C. Cherkin, K. Saunders, V. M. Gonzalez , D. Laurent, C. Rutter, and F. Comite. 1998. A randomized trial of a lay person-led self-management group intervention for back pain patients in primary care. *Spine* 23 (23):2608-51.

Veterans Administration. 2001a. "Enrollment in VA's Health Care System: Eligibility." Online. Available at http://www.va.gov/health/elig/eligibility.html [accessed May 3, 2001a].

———. 2001b. "Facts about the Department of Veterans Affairs." Online. Available at http://www.va.gov/pressrel/vafact01.htm [accessed Apr. 3, 2002b].

Von Korff, M., J. Gruman, J. Schaefer, S. Curry, and E. Wagner. 1997. Collaborative management of chronic illness. *Ann Intern Med* 127 (1097-1102).

Wagner, E., B. Austin, and M. Von Korff. 1996. Organizing care for patients with chronic illness. *Milbank Q* 74 (4):511-42.

Wagner, E. H., B. T. Austin, C. Davis, M. Hindmarsh, J. Schaefer, and A. Bonomi. 2001. Improving chronic illness care: translating evidence into action. *Health Aff (Millwood)* 20 (6):64-78.

Westmoreland, T., Federal Legislation Clinic of Georgetown University Law Center, Prepared for The Henry J. Kaiser Family Foundation. 1999. "KFF: Medicaid and HIV/AIDS Policy: A Basic Primer (pdf)." Online. Available at http://www.kff.org/content/1999/2136/1891-KFF.pdf [accessed Apr. 1, 2002].

Wood, D. L. (Chair, Secretary's Advisory Committee on Regulatory Reform). 10 August 2002. Final Report, to be issued in October 2002. Personal communication to Janet Corrigan.

Young, A. S., R. Klap, C. D. Sherbourne, and K. B. Wells. 2001. The quality of care for depressive and anxiety disorders in the United States. *Arch Gen Psychiatry* 58 (1):55-61.

3

Coordinating the Roles of the Federal Government to Enhance Quality of Care

Summary of Chapter Recommendations

The federal government has the central role in shaping all aspects of the health care sector. Strong federal leadership, a clear direction in pursuit of common aims, and consistent policies and practices across all government health care functions and programs are needed to raise the level of quality for the programs' beneficiaries and to drive improvement in the health care sector overall.

RECOMMENDATION 2: The federal government should take maximal advantage of its unique position as regulator, health care purchaser, health care provider, and sponsor of applied health services research to set quality standards for the health care sector. Specifically:

a. Regulatory processes should be used to establish clinical data reporting requirements applicable to all six major government health care programs.

b. All six major government health care programs should vigorously pursue purchasing strategies that encourage the adoption of best practices through the release of public domain comparative quality data and the provision of financial and other rewards to providers that achieve high levels of quality.

c. Not only should health care delivery systems operated by the public programs continue to serve as laboratories for the development of innovative 21st-century care delivery models, but much greater emphasis should be placed on the dissemination of findings and, in the case of information technology, the creation of public-domain products.

d. Applied health services research should be expanded and should emphasize the development of knowledge, tools, and strategies that can support quality enhancement in a wide variety of settings.

OVERVIEW OF FEDERAL ROLES

The federal government plays a number of different roles in the American health care arena, including regulator; purchaser of care; provider of health care services; and sponsor of applied research, demonstrations, and education and training programs for health care professionals. Each of these roles can support the accomplishment of somewhat different objectives along the spectrum from quality assurance to quality improvement to quality innovation.

As discussed in Chapter 1, research demonstrates wide variability in the quality of health care. As illustrated in Figure 3-1, some proportion of care is poor and unsafe; no patient should be exposed to this care. Some care is adequate, but not as good as it should be. Most of the services received by patients are effective, but the benefits are not as great as they could be, and resource use is unnecessarily high. Some fraction of patients receive very good care that is consistent with best practices, and an even smaller fraction probably receives excellent care employing state-of-the-art practices. Efforts to improve quality seek to shift the curve to the right and to truncate the left tail of the distribution.

It is through its regulator role that the federal government establishes minimal health care standards. Effective regulatory requirements protect beneficiaries from incompetent, impaired, and inadequately trained clinicians and from health care organizations that lack the requisite capabilities and processes to provide a minimal level of quality. Although regulatory "floors" can continually be raised, thus tightening the distribution of services by quality, regulatory approaches most often seek to cull substandard providers—to truncate the left tail of the distribution. Regulatory requirements have generally been set at levels that nearly all providers could satisfy. Regulatory requirements can have adverse impacts as well, by creating unnecessary reporting burdens, conveying conflicting objectives, and omitting essential elements of quality.

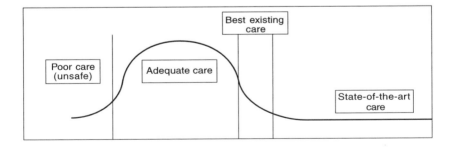

FIGURE 3-1 Distribution of care by level of quality, a conceptual scheme.

Although the federal government has for decades relied extensively on regulatory strategies to address quality concerns, there has been considerable evolution in the types of regulatory requirements. Traditionally, regulatory requirements focused on *quality assurance*—structural or competency requirements for hospitals (e.g., all hospitals must have well-defined infection control processes) or health care professionals (e.g., physicians and nurses must attain a given level of training and maintain current state licenses). Over decades, regulatory strategies, especially those applicable to the government programs that deliver care through the private sector (i.e., Medicare, Medicaid, and the State Children's Health Insurance Program [SCHIP]), have incorporated *quality improvement* approaches that focus more on demonstrating improvement in care processes and patient outcomes. For example, Medicare+Choice (M+C) health plans must collect data on specific performance measures and demonstrate improvement over time. Regulatory strategies that focus on quality improvement offer some potential to shift the quality distribution to the right, although very little is known about which of these approaches works best.

It is this transition from quality assurance to quality improvement strategies that has also broadened the potential for the government to strengthen its roles as purchaser and health care provider. Quality improvement strategies emphasize direct measurement of the clinical quality of care and of patient perceptions and outcomes, and these data then enable differentiation of various levels of quality.

In its purchaser role, the government could reward providers that achieve high levels of quality. Purchasing strategies can raise the quality of care provided by the majority of providers thus shifting the curve to the right. Such strategies include public disclosure of comparative quality data on providers and health plans, and financial and other rewards for high levels of quality.

The disclosure of comparative performance data on hospitals, health plans, physicians, and other providers draws attention to best practices in hopes of encouraging other providers to adopt them. To the extent that consumers act on this information when making choices, health care providers have incentives to improve their performance, thus increasing demand for their services and their market share. Public disclosure of comparative quality data may spur action on the part of providers themselves or professional groups, with steps being taken to encourage poor performers to enhance their knowledge and skills or limit the scope of their practice. Furthermore, public disclosure may stimulate public support for the exercising of regulatory authority by federal or state governments to address persistent poor performance.

The purchaser role also relies on linkages between payment and performance. The federal government (acting on behalf of program benefi-ciaries) might engage in selective contracting with the highest-quality pro-viders. Providers (e.g., hospitals, physicians, and plans) that achieved ex-emplary performance might receive higher fees, diagnosis related group (DRG) payments, capitation rates, or bonuses. Proper risk adjustment (see Chapter 2) is critical to payment strategies that reward quality, as public recognition also attracts patients with more complex care needs.

In its provider role, the federal government assumes all the responsi-bilities of ownership of health care institutions, employer of the health care workforce, and manager and operator of comprehensive delivery systems. In this capacity, it has an opportunity to serve as a laboratory in which to test new financing, delivery, and information dissemination models, while experimenting with various quality measurement and im-provement strategies. Just as performance measurement activities have proliferated within the regulatory requirements for Medicare, Medicaid, and SCHIP, performance measurement and improvement have become an integral component of the clinical management processes of the Veter-ans Health Administration (VHA), Department of Defense (DOD) TRICARE, and Indian Health Service (IHS) programs. As discussed in Chapter 5, VHA and DOD have also led the way in building clinical infor-mation systems to support care delivery, quality improvement, patient safety, surveillance and monitoring, and many other applications.

As a major sponsor of applied health services research, the federal government provides support for the development of the knowledge and creation of the tools needed to carry out more effectively the regulator, purchaser, and health care delivery roles. In recent years, the focus of state of the art quality enhancement has shifted toward the measurement of clinical quality (i.e., medical care processes and outcomes) and con-sumer perceptions. Through the Agency for Healthcare Research and Quality (AHRQ) and other applied research programs sponsored by the National Institutes of Health (NIH), VHA, the Food and Drug Adminis-tration, and the Centers for Disease Control and Prevention, the federal government can assist in the development of quality measures, survey instruments, and public reporting tools to enhance federal and state regu-latory functions and public and private purchasing activities. The federal government also supports applied health services research that addresses many of the broader health care financing and delivery issues important to creating an environment that supports quality. For example, AHRQ conducts applied research and demonstrations on payment approaches and quality incentives, health care delivery models, and clinical decision-support systems.

The committee recognizes that the federal government influences the health care sector in numerous other ways that are outside the immediate scope of this project. NIH provides extensive support for clinical research designed to expand the scientific knowledge base and develop new medical technology. The federal government provides extensive support for the education and training of health care professionals, and these programs offer yet another opportunity for the federal government to influence quality and safety. The Medicare program provides about two-thirds of the approximately $18 billion spent annually to educate medical residents (Anderson et al., 2001). In fiscal year 2001, the Bureau of Health Professions and the Bureau of Primary Health Care devoted about $460 million to health professions training, including physicians, nurses, dentists, allied health professionals, and public health practitioners (MedPAC, 2001). NIH provides support for the training of researchers through a variety of mechanisms (Association of American Medical Colleges, 2001). The federal and state governments provide further support for the health care sector through tax policy, including the exclusion of employers' contributions to group health insurance from taxable income for employees, granting of tax exempt status to many health care institutions, and individual tax deductions for certain health care expenditures (Arnett, 1999).

This chapter is not intended to provide a comprehensive assessment of all of these government roles, but rather a focused review of how the government might better employ some of them in carrying out quality enhancement processes. Specifically, the remainder of this chapter examines some of the ways in which the government health care programs could employ regulatory, purchasing, and care delivery strategies in their quality enhancement processes. Current efforts to standardize and coordinate those processes across the six programs are reviewed, and an overall approach to quality enhancement that maximally leverages the various government roles is outlined. Chapter 6 provides a discussion of the role of applied health services research in strengthening quality enhancement processes.

REGULATORY STRATEGIES

Each of the government health care programs has pursued a regulatory approach to some degree. In general, the programs that pay for services provided through the private sector (i.e., Medicare, Medicaid, SCHIP, and DOD TRICARE) rely more on regulatory approaches than do those that provide most services directly through government-owned provider organizations (i.e., VHA, DOD TRICARE, and IHS). The latter programs have the option of encouraging quality improvement through internal quality management activities (see the discussion of the government's care delivery role below).

All government programs rely to some extent on a patchwork of both federal and state laws and enforcement programs that are intertwined. Historically, state laws have established certain requirements for the licensing of clinicians and institutional providers, and form the bedrock of the regulatory system. Layered over state laws are various federal regulatory requirements, many of which are tied to state or local law.

A sizable body of federal regulatory requirements pertaining to Medicare and, to a lesser degree, Medicaid has slowly but steadily accumulated over the years (American Hospital Association, 2002). It is through these two government programs, which contract with the majority of private providers, that the federal government has the greatest impact on the nation's health care delivery system. Other government health care programs tend to apply many of Medicare's regulatory requirements.

In most government programs, regulatory standards focus on institutional providers, clinicians, and health plans that seek to receive payment from or deliver care under an identified program (see Tables 3-1 and 3-2). In the Medicaid and SCHIP programs, however, regulatory requirements are the responsibility of the state governments that administer the programs, and it is the responsibility of the state to ensure that providers and health plans satisfy federal requirements.

In general, regulatory standards fall into two groups—standards of participation and external review processes—although the lines of distinction are not always clear. Most standards of participation are aimed at ensuring that providers have and/or maintain certain key competencies, while external review refers to the assessment of provider performance (e.g., care processes and patient outcomes) by an independent organization, usually a quality improvement organization (QIO).

Standards for Participation

A good deal of the regulation in each government program's portfolio is intended to ensure that program participants possess minimal levels of competence and comply with health and safety requirements. For institutions, these include requirements pertaining to physical safety and sanitation, as well as such organizational competencies as governance, internal quality review, credentialing of medical staff, and medical records management.

Typically, these minimal participatory standards require compliance with state and local licensing laws as a threshold requirement for participation, with some variations. In the DOD TRICARE and IHS programs, clinicians can be licensed in any one of the states. In addition to licensure, most clinicians must comply with state scope-of-practice rules. Such rules are an important determinant of (1) the availability and choice of clinicians (e.g., a broad scope-of-practice for nonphysician providers increases

TABLE 3-1 Overview of Regulatory Requirements in Medicare, Medicaid, and SCHIP

	MEDICARE		MEDICAID		SCHIP
	Fee-for-Service (FFS)	Managed Care	Medicaid FFS	Medicaid Managed Care[a]	
Target entities	Institutional providers and clinicians that receive Medicare reimbursement.	Medicare+Choice plans	Institutional providers and clinicians that receive Medicaid reimbursement	State Medicaid programs and managed care plans that enroll Medicaid beneficiaries	State SCHIP programs
Requirements	Must meet standards for physical structure, governance, quality assurance, staff credentialing, infection control, etc. Participation in external review projects is voluntary; other health care institutions must respond to data requests from QIOs.	Must implement a quality improvement process and show results using the Medicare HEDIS, CAHPS, and the Health Outcomes Survey. Participation in external review is mandatory.	Medicare rules apply for institutional providers.	The Medicaid program must ensure that managed care plans use a quality improvement process that collects, assesses, and reports performance data to clinicians. States must contract with an EQRO[b] for annual quality reviews and conduct annual medical audits of each managed care contractor.	The State Child Health Plan must describe performance goals; how progress will be assessed; and assure CMS that the state will collect, assess, and report standardized data. External review requirements are at states' discretion.

Enforcement	CMS contracts with state agencies to conduct certification surveys of hospitals, nursing facilities, home health agencies, and other providers. JCAHO has deeming authority for hospitals, ambulatory surgical centers, clinical laboratories, home health agencies, and hospices. Failure to comply can lead to sanctions or cutoff of Medicare payments.	Failure to comply with CMS rules disqualifies M+C plans from enrolling Medicare beneficiaries. NCQA has deeming authority for managed care plans or quality assurance, antidiscrimination, access to services, enrollee records, advance directives, and provider participation rules.	CMS contracts with state agencies to conduct surveys of hospitals, nursing facilities, home health agencies, and other providers. JCAHO has deeming authority in many states. Failure to comply can lead to sanctions or cutoff of Medicaid payments.	Failure to comply can result in disallowance of federal financial participation in contract payments to managed care organizations. Failure to meet the Medicaid waiver conditions can lead to nonrenewal or termination of waiver or a "compliance enforcement action."	CMS reviews SCHIP programs by analyzing the state's policies and procedures, conducting on-site reviews, and reviewing samples of individual case records. Failure to comply can result in disallowance of federal financial participation. External review has not been applied in most free-standing programs.

*a*The Balanced Budget Act (BBA) of 1997 (P.L. 105-33, Sec. 4705) will significantly change quality improvement in Medicaid when implemented. The legislation calls for extensive state efforts to improve quality and to provide for external, independent review of Medicaid managed care. The final rules implementing the Medicaid managed care provisions were released after the committee completed deliberations. This table reflects the rules in effect at the time of review.

*b*EQROs may be QIOs, other entities that meet federal QIO requirements, or private accreditation bodies.

SOURCES: Health Care Financing Administration, n.d., 1998, 2000; MedPAC, 2002; and 42 Code of Federal Regulations §434.34; §457.200.

TABLE 3-2 Overview of Regulatory Requirements: VHA, DOD
TRICARE, and IHS

	VHA	DOD TRICARE	IHS
Target entities	Institutional providers and clinicians that provide care to VHA beneficiaries	Institutional providers, clinicians, and networks that serve TRICARE beneficiaries	IHS-funded institutional providers and clinicians
Requirements	VHA hospitals, facilities, and other providers must be accredited by JCAHO or some other accrediting group. Clinicians must be credentialed according to VHA policies and JCAHO standards. An external review program covers all VHA facilities. The current contractor is the West Virginia Medical Institute, Inc.	Institutional providers, clinicians, and networks must be Medicare-approved (where relevant). Except for operational ambulatory clinics (treating active-duty personnel only), all "fixed" hospitals and freestanding ambulatory clinics must be accredited by JCAHO or some other applicable accrediting group A national external review program is carried out by KePRO, Inc.	Most IHS facilities are accredited by JCAHO or the Accreditation Association for Ambulatory Health (AAAHC), or certified by CMS (whichever is relevant). Must meet the external review requirements of the Medicare and Medicaid programs.
Enforcement	Failure to comply disqualifies clinicians from serving VHA beneficiaries. Deficiencies in compliance generally lead to corrective action initiatives.	Failure to meet the quality standards and certification requirements may result in termination of payments and identification as a non-authorized provider.	Deficiencies in compliance generally lead to corrective action initiatives.

SOURCES: Department of Defense, 1995, 2001; Indian Health Service, 2001b; Pittman, 2002; and Veterans Administration, 2001.

the supply of primary care providers); (2) the degree of interdependence and authority of various types of health care professionals (Cooper et al., 1998); (3) the ability to deliver care through multidisciplinary teams (e.g., proscriptive state scope-of-practice acts limit innovation in redefining roles and functions performed by nonphysician health care professionals) (Sage and Aiken, 1997); and (4) the development of approaches to care delivery and organization that cross state lines (e.g., provision of care through use of the Internet and multistate provider groups) (Finocchio et al., 1998; Rosenfeld et al., 2000; Sage and Aiken, 1997). Participation standards reflect a good deal of consistency among programs. Most of the federal programs require that providers conform to Medicare standards of participation, but there are some exceptions. For example, SCHIP programs that do not operate as Medicaid expansions are required to conform only to state-established standards of participation.

Enforcement of compliance is generally delegated to a web of private organizations and state agencies that conduct inspections and certify that standards have been met. The Joint Commission on Accreditation of Healthcare Organizations (JCAHO) has statutory authority under Medicare to certify hospitals, ambulatory surgical centers, clinical laboratories, home health agencies, and hospices as being in compliance with federal regulations. This authority is based on the concept that organizations meeting JCAHO standards are "deemed" to meet federal standards. The Centers for Medicare and Medicaid Services (CMS) is required to monitor the performance of JCAHO, as well as that of other organizations with deemed status to ensure that equivalency is maintained. JCAHO accreditation is also accepted in the VHA, DOD TRICARE, and IHS programs. The National Committee for Quality Assurance (NCQA) was recently granted deeming authority for certain requirements pertaining to M+C plans and has similar authority for health plans in TRICARE and in some states for Medicaid (NCQA, 2002). Deeming is one way to reduce the burden of repetitive inspections, but there must be adequate oversight to ensure that accrediting entities carry out this responsibility properly (MedPAC, 2000).

Very little work has been done to assess the effect of conditions of participation, as currently structured and enforced, on processes of care or patient outcomes. In addition, the minimal standards are updated infrequently, and little evaluation is done to streamline standards to ensure that they focus on requirements that actually improve patient safety and quality of care (MedPAC, 2000).

External Review

External review is used most extensively by Medicare and Medicaid. External review under Medicare started in the early 1970s,[1] and is currently carried out by a network of 37 private-sector QIOs (formerly known as peer review organizations), under contract with CMS. Other govern-

---

[1]Social Security Amendments of 1972 (P.L. 92-603).

ment programs, state governments, and private-sector groups also contract with QIOs. External review focuses on measurement of care processes and patient outcomes through such means as abstraction of samples of medical records (conducted by QIO staff or the providers); screening of hospital discharge abstracts and claims data to identify such events as nosocomial infections, unscheduled returns to surgery, and deaths; and conduct of a wealth of focused studies in selected clinical areas (discussed further in Chapter 4).

Under Medicare fee-for-service (FFS), QIO review is mandatory for hospitals and other institutions, and there are some QIO activities for ambulatory care in which physicians may voluntarily choose to participate. Starting in 1985, quality review (by QIOs or QIO-like entities) became mandatory for health plans (Consolidated Omnibus Budget Resolution Act [COBRA] 1985); today, the review processes for M+C plans are more extensive than those conducted for FFS Medicare.

During the late 1970s and 1980s, quality review programs were developed and applied within state Medicaid programs. These efforts are difficult to characterize because federal quality requirements and activities differ by type of health care program, which include FFS programs, primary care case management programs, capitated full-risk managed care, Section 1915(b) waiver programs, Section 1115 waiver demonstrations, home and community-based services waiver programs, and programs of all-inclusive care for elderly beneficiaries (Shalala, 2000).

Federal law pertaining to the Medicaid program requires that states adopt procedures to evaluate the utilization of care and services and establish a plan for reviewing the appropriateness and quality of care. The federal government pays states an enhanced federal financial participation rate of 75 percent (as opposed to an average closer to 50 percent) to help cover the costs of reviews conducted by QIOs or QIO-like entities, and most states have pursued this option (Verdier and Dodge, 2002). States, however, have considerable latitude in how they choose to define, implement, and enforce quality review; the level and degree of external review vary widely among the states.

With the growth of Medicare and Medicaid managed care options in the 1990s and in response to concerns about burden and conflicting quality requirements, CMS developed the Quality Improvement System for Managed Care (QISMC), which is based on technical performance measurement (Centers for Medicare and Medicaid Services, 2001a). The system is mandatory for M+C plans and voluntary for Medicaid managed care. QISMC relies to a great extent on measures in the Health Plan Employer Data and Information Set (HEDIS); the standardized quality measurement set of the NCQA; and the Consumer Assessment of Health Plans (CAHPS), a survey instrument and reporting system developed to help consumers and purchasers choose among health plans (see Chapters 4 and 6). QISMC also includes fairly extensive requirements pertaining to the internal quality assurance and improvement processes of health plans.

In addition to Medicare and Medicaid, other government health care programs rely to varying degrees on external review to safeguard quality. The DOD TRICARE program contracts with the Keystone Peer Review Organization to review the appropriateness of care for about 1,500 medical, surgical, and mental health cases per month; to certify mental health facilities; and to handle patient and provider appeals. VHA has traditional regulatory programs, including an external peer review program. But in these government programs that own and operate their own delivery systems, external review activities are overshadowed by the quality management and improvement programs embedded in the health care delivery function (discussed below) (Institute of Medicine, 2001c).

While external review in all the programs relies on performance measurement of various types to assess the quality of care being delivered, these assessments are necessarily limited by the absence of supportive tools and infrastructure. In the absence of computer-based record keeping on elements of care, quality-of-care studies are confined to manual extractions from paper medical records, resulting in time-consuming analysis of small samples, or to the sparse clinical information available on claims. Moreover, the lack of consistent standards among states and review organizations, the lack of consistent datasets, and the inadequacy of the data in general create substantial obstacles to establishing quality benchmarks or making valid cross-program comparisons of the quality of care received. As discussed in Chapter 5, some progress has been made in addressing these issues in recent years, but the pace of progress is too slow in light of the gravity of the quality and safety shortcomings.

PURCHASING STRATEGIES

There have been very few attempts to expand upon traditional purchasing regulatory mechanisms and engage in what is called "value-based purchasing." Two different strategies are at the heart of value-based purchasing: (1) disclosure of comparative quality information to encourage consumers and purchasers to choose the highest-quality providers, and (2) selective purchasing or payment incentives to providers and beneficiaries. The purpose of value-based purchasing is to promote market forces that encourage and reward (through higher market share and/or higher payments) providers that achieve higher levels of quality. Both information disclosure and payment incentives, however, are dependent upon the availability of comparative quality data on providers and few such data are available. Moreover, some comparisons of performance require risk adjustment for differences in patient mix. Such comparisons, too, require richer clinical information than is currently available in most administrative datasets.

In the Medicare program, the federal government has taken some steps consistent with its purchaser role by facilitating disclosure of comparative quality data in the public domain. In 1998, the National Medicare Education Program—an initiative to educate beneficiaries about Medicare health care options—was launched. Under this program, CMS makes available on the World Wide Web limited comparative quality data for M+C plans from CAHPS and HEDIS to help beneficiaries select an M+C plan. For the nearly 87 percent of beneficiaries enrolled in Medicare FFS, the primary decisions to be made are whether to shift from FFS to an M+C plan and what clinician to select. Current information does not permit a comparison to support the former decision, because most performance data are available only for M+C plans. Few if any performance data are available to help beneficiaries choose a doctor or other clinician.

CMS provides beneficiaries with comparative data on kidney dialysis centers, as required by the Balanced Budget Act of 1998. CMS funded the development of clinical practice measures, based on the practice guidelines of the National Kidney Foundation's Dialysis Outcome Quality Initiative and awarded the development contract to Pro-West (Centers for Medicare and Medicaid Services, 2001c). The measures were developed collaboratively with providers, and dialysis facilities were given the opportunity to review their data prior to public release (American Association of Kidney Patients, 2001). There is a strong commitment to public disclosure, and the CMS website provides a rating of dialysis centers as average, below average, or above average (Centers for Medicare and Medicaid Services, 2002a). CMS recently announced its intent to make similar comparative quality information available on nursing homes. Data from a pilot project conducted in six states (Colorado, Florida, Maryland, Ohio, Rhode Island, and Washington) using the Minimum Data Set measures were recently released (Centers for Medicare and Medicaid Services, 2001b).

At present, CMS has very limited authority to link payment to performance for traditional Medicare, other than through demonstration projects designed to test alternative purchasing approaches (MedPAC, 1999). For example, under the Centers of Excellence demonstration, Medicare contracts selectively with a limited number of hospitals or other organizations to provide comprehensive services for specific procedures (e.g., heart transplants, total joint replacement procedures) under a bundled payment scheme (Centers for Medicare and Medicaid Services, 2002b). Providers compete for these contracts on the basis of quality, as well as other factors, such as geographic accessibility, organizational capacity, and price. CMS is also conducting disease management demonstration projects that focus on Medicare FFS beneficiaries with congestive heart failure, diabetes, and coronary heart disease. These demonstrations involve innovative care management approaches, expanded coverage for prescription drugs, and the assumption of financial risk by providers (Centers for Medicare and Medicaid Services, 2002c). In addition, CMS has awarded 15 grants for coordinated care demonstration projects focused on Medicare fee-for-service beneficiaries with complex chronic conditions, and these, too, involve care delivery innovations and alternative payment models (Department of Health and Human Services, 2001).

In 1997, DOD initiated a Centers of Excellence program to select, on the basis of a rigorous evaluation process, a limited number of providers to deliver highly specialized services in selected clinical areas (TRICARE, 2002). This program is not yet operational, but a great deal of work has been done to identify the selected clinical areas and the criteria for selection. The selected areas are bone marrow and solid organ transplants, burn care, cardiac care, complex general surgery, cranial and spinal procedures, gynecologic oncology, head and neck oncology, neonatal and prenatal medicine, and total joint replacement. The criteria for selection emphasize the ability to measure various aspects of quality, adjust for severity, measure outcomes, and report externally on clinical processes and outcomes.

In 1998, DOD began reporting some information on quality and access to beneficiaries (Department of Defense, 2001). The Military Treatment Facility Report Card includes information on waiting times for major services; patient satisfaction; and summary scores from JCAHO accreditation surveys applicable to credentialing, provider/staff competence, infection control, and nursing care.

Although beyond the immediate scope of the present study, it should be noted that the federal government has pursued a purchaser approach in carrying out its responsibilities under the Federal Employees Health Benefits Program. For health plans participating in this program, federal employees can access CAHPS and HEDIS data and summary results from NCQA accreditation surveys (Office of Personnel Management, 2002).

CARE DELIVERY

VHA and IHS have comprehensive care delivery programs. For the most part, the federal government owns and operates the health care facilities and employs the workforce necessary to provide comprehensive services to beneficiaries in these programs. The DOD TRICARE program also has a large delivery system component—just over half of health care services are provided through DOD's treatment facilities (located mainly on military bases), with the remainder being delivered through private-sector providers. Each of these government programs has pursued a variety of quality measurement and improvement activities as an integral part of its quality management activities (see Table 3-3).

The VHA program stands apart from most health care programs, both public and private, in its commitment to building the strong organizational supports necessary to provide safe and effective care. In the late 1970s, VHA recognized the important role of clinical decision-support systems in improving quality. During the 1980s and 1990s, VHA created the Veterans Health Information Systems and Technology Architecture (VistA), a computerized patient records system that now extends throughout all 1,100 VHA facilities (including 172 hospitals) in the United States (Institute of Medicine, 2001c). Since 1997, VHA has taken steps to make the automated clinical information more accessible and meaningful at the point of care (see Chapter 5).

VistA serves as the foundation for an extensive program of quality measurement and improvement and clinical decision support, including ongoing benchmarking across a wide range of preventive, acute, and chronic care quality measures; automated entry of medication orders; a notification system that alerts clinicians about clinically significant events identified through the use of integrated laboratory, radiology, pharmacy, progress notes, and other data; a clinical reminder system to promote evidence-based practice; and use of bar codes for medication administration and verification of blood type prior to transfusion.

The DOD TRICARE program conducts numerous quality measurement and improvement projects, including ones that use the HEDIS measurement set and beneficiary surveys such as CAHPS. In recent years, DOD has made progress in developing a computerized clinical information system (see Chapter 5). IHS has emphasized improving diabetes care across the various regions using a standardized measurement set.

CURRENT EFFORTS TO STANDARDIZE AND COORDINATE

Important efforts have been made in recent years to coordinate the quality enhancement activities of the various government health care programs. AHRQ has played a central role in many of these efforts. Its contribution to the development of CAHPS and other standardized tools and techniques for quality measurement and improvement is noteworthy. CAHPS is now used by DOD TRICARE, state Medicaid agencies, private-sector purchasers (e.g., Ford Motor Company, Vermont Employer's Health Care Alliance), Federal Employees Health Benefit Program (FEHBP), and accrediting bodies (e.g., NCQA) (Agency for Healthcare Research and Quality, 2000). To facilitate widespread use and public disclosure of comparative results, AHRQ established a National CAHPS

TABLE 3-3 Internal Quality Management Activities: VHA, DOD TRICARE, and IHS

	VHA	DOD TRICARE	IHS
Target entities	Institutional providers, clinicians, and facilities that provide direct patient care to VHA beneficiaries	Institutional providers, clinicians, and networks that serve active duty military personnel and other DOD TRICARE beneficiaries	IHS providers, hospitals, health centers, and clinics
Internal Quality Management Activities	An internal Performance Measurement Program (QUERI), which evaluates in-house outcome measures as well as HEDIS and JCAHO measures adopted by the VHA external review contractor and other sources. Two patient surveys: the Veteran Satisfaction Survey and the American Consumer Satisfaction Index. The National Surgical Quality Improvement Program, an ongoing effort to evaluate and improve surgical outcomes. The National Center for Patient Safety, used for evaluating "close calls" and adverse events.	Numerous special quality studies, including ones that use HEDIS measures and various beneficiary satisfaction surveys	The Performance Evaluation System, which includes a patient database and information system for identifying health problems and needs among the IHS population. The Indian Health Diabetes Care and Outcomes Audit, which involves chart reviews to determine compliance with the IHS standards of care for diabetes.

SOURCES: Code of Federal Regulations, 2001; Department of Defense, 2001; Indian Health Service, 2000, 2001a; Institute of Medicine, 2001b; KePRO, 2001; Kizer, 1995; and Veterans Health Administration, 2001.

Benchmarking Database in which survey sponsors participate on a voluntary basis. The database currently includes data from over 900 health plans (Agency for Healthcare Research and Quality, 2001c).

AHRQ plays an important role in various interagency collaborative efforts. The agency is mandated by statute to provide coordination of quality improvement programs and activities among the various government health care programs. The primary vehicle for this purpose is the Quality Interagency Coordinating Committee (QuIC).[2] The QuIC was established in 1998 to ensure that all federal agencies involved in regulating, purchasing, providing, or studying health care services coordinate their activities with the common goal of improving quality. The membership of the QuIC includes representation from within the Department of Health and Human Services (DHHS) (i.e., CMS, IHS and AHRQ), DOD, VHA, and numerous other federal agencies (see Chapter 4). The QuIC has work groups on issues such as providing consumer information, measuring quality, improving clinical quality, developing the work force, and improving information systems (Agency for Healthcare Research and Quality, 2001a).

Lastly, AHRQ leads an interagency initiative started in 2000 to address patient safety concerns (Agency for Healthcare Research and Quality, 2001b). The Patient Safety Task Force includes representatives of AHRQ, CMS, the Centers for Disease Control and Prevention, and the Food and Drug Administration. The goals of the task force are to (1) coordinate the collection and analysis of safety-related data across various government programs; (2) exchange information on patient safety reporting and practices with other public-and private-sector initiatives; (3) disseminate analyses to health care providers and others; and (4) carry out research, programs, and projects that will improve patient safety.

LEVERAGING THE GOVERNMENT ROLES

There are, of course, important differences across the government health care programs in the roles played by the federal government and the degree of emphasis placed on any individual role in influencing qual-

---

[2]Healthcare Research and Quality Act of 1999, Title IX of the Public Health Service Act (42 U.S.C. 299 et seq.). The QuIC has enjoyed the support of many governmental health care programs. Its principal mission is to enable federal health care programs to coordinate their quality improvement activities. The QuIC's work is financially supported and staffed by the participating federal agencies—the Department of Commerce, Department of Defense, Department of Health and Human Services, Deartment of Labor, Federal Bureau of Prisons, Federal Trade Commission, National Highway Transportation Safety Administration, Office of Management and Budget, Office of Personnel Management, United States Coast Guard, and Veterans Administration.

ity. This is the case in part because the programs have very different historical underpinnings and statutory enabling authorities. In general, the programs vary in terms of the degree of responsibility the federal government assumes for quality; the political and other barriers to addressing quality concerns; and the incentives, tools, and data available to measure and improve quality.

On one end of the spectrum is Medicaid, in which the federal government has a very small role in quality enhancement. Federal regulatory requirements are minimal, and the states, which administer the program, have a great deal of latitude in carrying out quality oversight responsibilities. For the most part, both federal and state governments have pursued regulatory approaches to quality enhancement for the program.

On the other end of the spectrum are the federal health care delivery programs, such as the VHA, DOD TRICARE, and IHS programs. In these programs, the federal government assumes nearly total responsibility for quality. In these programs, there is less distinction, and certainly less conflict, among the various types of federal roles. In the case of VHA, and more recently DOD, the federal government has used its formidable influence and resources to build an information infrastructure capable of supporting a wide range of quality measurement, clinical decision-support, and care delivery applications. The accomplishments of these programs represent best practices that the federal government should actively share with other public- and private-sector health care programs.

Somewhere in the middle of this spectrum is Medicare. Established as a traditional indemnity insurance program, Medicare has emphasized the use of regulatory mechanisms to protect beneficiaries from poor-quality providers. The transition to producing comparative quality data has been a gradual one, and attempts at public disclosure of these data have been sporadic and infrequent.

There is little doubt that the federal government could play its various roles more effectively to both promote improvements in quality within each of the government health care programs and drive improvement in the health care sector overall. The federal government should exercise appropriate influence through *each* of its roles to the maximum extent possible to promote quality improvements. Specifically, the committee encourages the leadership of the various government health care programs to ensure that their quality enhancement processes adhere to the following guiding principles:

1. *Government health care programs should establish consistent quality expectations and requirements and apply them fairly and equitably to all financing and delivery options within a program.*
2. *Government health care programs should promote and encourage provid-*

ers to strive for excellence by providing financial and other rewards and public recognition to providers who achieve superior levels of quality.

3. Government health care programs should actively collaborate with each other and private-sector quality enhancement organizations with regard to all aspects of quality enhancement—including use of standardized measures and sharing of data—where doing so will likely result in greater gains in quality or reduced provider burden.

4. Government health care programs should encourage and enable active consumer participation in efforts to enhance quality through such means as the following:

> *a.   Raising consumer awareness of the magnitude of quality and safety shortcomings and the means of addressing these problems*
>
> *b.   Seeking consumer input into the design and evaluation of quality enhancement processes*
>
> *c.   Including patient assessments of quality and service in the portfolio of performance measures*
>
> *d.   Providing patients with health information necessary to evaluate treatment options and participate in care management*
>
> *e.   Providing consumers with comparative performance data on providers and health plans*

5. Government health care programs, in collaboration with the Agency for Healthcare Research and Quality (AHRQ), should pursue a rich agenda of applied research and demonstrations focusing on tools, techniques, and approaches to quality enhancement.

There are many variations in quality enhancement requirements across the government health care programs, some rooted in differences among the needs of the populations served, but most stemming from the fact that the programs have developed their quality enhancement processes independently. In the absence of compelling reasons for differences in quality enhancement requirements, the federal government should strive to provide the same minimal level of quality protection to all populations served. Efforts should also be made to streamline the implementation of quality enhancement processes so as to minimize the burden on providers, especially those in the private sector, who typically have relationships with multiple third-party payers.

The federal government has far less experience in pursuing purchasing strategies to enhance quality than in establishing regulatory requirements. Given the seriousness of current safety and quality shortcomings in the health care system, it is imperative that the government be given the flexibility and resources necessary to explore value-based purchasing. Regulations alone cannot solve the problem. Purchasing initiatives should be carefully evaluated to determine whether they are effective. Purchasing strategies should be aimed at creating an environment that will encourage and reward exemplary performance. Purchasing strategies are less rigid than regulatory requirements, and their expected effects are more difficult to predict and to quantify. Yet such strategies have the potential to motivate the majority of health care providers to improve quality, thus encouraging widespread change in the health care sector that would complement regulatory efforts.

One purchasing strategy—public disclosure of comparative quality data on providers—also has the potential to engage numerous other stakeholders in the quality debate. Government health care programs provide little if any information to the public on variations in quality and outcomes across hospitals, provider groups, and treatment programs; yet, there is a strong evidence base to substantiate that such variations are large (Schuster et al., 1998). Not all beneficiaries are capable of or interested in incorporating information on quality into their decisions when selecting providers or treatment programs, but not all need do so to provide incentives to improve performance. Other stakeholders, including group purchasers, professional leaders, governing boards of hospitals and other institutions, peer review organizations, and state and federal regulators would find comparative quality data useful in carrying out their responsibilities.

Finally, the federal government must provide leadership for the development of the infrastructure needed to support quality oversight and improvement. All of the federal health care programs have made a stronger commitment in recent years to technical quality measurement. Nearly all of the programs have focused a good deal of attention on quality measures pertaining to leading chronic conditions in response to the needs of the populations they serve. The increased emphasis on clinical quality measurement in all of the federal health care programs is a positive development, highlighting the potential for the federal government to encourage greater coordination and standardization of performance measurement efforts across government programs and, indeed, throughout the health care sector overall. In the absence of strong federal leadership and a clear strategy for coordinating the efforts of various government health care programs, the likely outcome will be a duplicative and burdensome patchwork of quality measurement data of limited utility to end users (as discussed further in Chapter 4).

In general, there is a lack of recognition of the dependence of effective quality oversight and improvement efforts on computerized clinical data (as discussed further in Chapter 5). Despite numerous reports in recent years calling attention to the importance of computerized clinical data (Institute of Medicine, 2001a; National Committee for Quality Assurance,

2002), the development of an information technology infrastructure to support quality enhancement processes has been very slow.

The challenge for federal quality enhancement processes is to harness their potential to drive and facilitate quality improvement throughout the health care delivery system. Without coordination, standardization, dissemination of information, and incentives, fulfillment of that potential will be impossible to attain.

REFERENCES

Agency for Healthcare Research and Quality. 2000. "CAHPS-User Story: AHRQ Publication No 00-P023." Online. Available at http://www.ahrq.gov/qual/cahps/cahpuser.htm [accessed May 6, 2002].

———. 2001a. "Quality Interagency Coordination Task Force (QuIC) Fact Sheet, AHRQ publication No. 00-P027." Online. Available at http://www.ahcpr.gov/qual/quicfact. htm [accessed June 18, 2001a].

———. 2001b. "Patient Safety Task Force Fact Sheet." Online. Available at http://www. ahrq.gov/qual/taskforce/psfactst.htm [accessed May 20, 2001b].

———. 2001c. "Annual Report of the National CAHPS ® Benchmarking Database 2000:What Consumers Say About the Quality of Their Health Plans and Medical Care." Online. Available at http://ncbd.cahps.org/pdf/NCBD2000AnRpt.pdf [accessed May 6, 2002c].

American Association of Kidney Patients. 2001. "What's new at HCFA." Online [accessed Aug. 14, 2002].

American Hospital Association. 2002. *Patients or Paperwork? The Regulatory Burden Facing America's Hospitals.* Washington DC: PricewaterhouseCoopers for American Hospital Association.

Anderson, G. F., G. D. Greenberg, and B. O. Wynn. 2001. Graduate Medical Education: The Policy Debate. *Annu Rev Public Health* 22:35-47.

Arnett, G-M. 1999. *Emporwering Health Care Consumers Through Tax Reform.* An Arbor MI: The University of Michigan Press.

Association of American Medical Colleges. 2001. AAMC Data Book: Statistical Information Related to Medical Schools and Teaching Hospitals. 102.

Centers for Medicare and Medicaid Services. 2001a. Medicaid Program, Medicaid Managed Care. Final Rule. Federal Register.

———. 2001b. "Nursing Home Compare - Home." Online. Available at http://www. medicare.gov/NHCompare/home.asp [accessed May 6, 2002b].

———. 2001c. "Quality of Care ~ National Projects, ESRD Clinical Performance Measures Project (2000 Annual Report)." Online. Available at hcfa.gov/quality/3m8.htm [accessed Jan. 9, 2002c].

———. 2002a. "Medicare.gov - Dialysis Facility Compare Home." Online. Available at http://www.medicare.gov/Dialysis/Home.asp [accessed Aug. 14, 2002a].

———. 2002b. "Medicare Partnerships for Quality Services Demonstration." Online. Available at http://cms.hhs.gov/healthplans/research/mpqsdem.asp [accessed Oct. 14, 2002b].

———. 2002c. Medicare Program; Solicitation for proposals for the demonstration project for disease management for severely chronically ill Medicare beneficiaries with congestive heart failure, diabetes, and coronary heart disease: Notice for Solicitation of Proposals. *Fed Regist* 67 (36):8267-70.

Code of Federal Regulations. 2001. "32CFR199.15: Quality and Utilization Review Peer Review Organization Program." Online. Available at http://www.tricare.osd.mil/CFR/C15.PDF [accessed May 9, 2002].

Cooper, R., T. Henderson, and C. Dietrich. 1998. Roles of Non-physician Clinicians as Autonomous Providers of Patient Care. *JAMA* 280 (9):795-802.

Department of Defense. 1995. *DoD Directive Number 6025.13 (July 20): Clinical Quality Management Program (CQMP) in the Military Health Services System (MHSS).*

———. 2001. "Healthcare Quality Initiatives Review Panel (HQIRP) Report." Online. Available at http://www.tricare.osd.mil/downloads/FinalReport123.pdf [accessed June 26, 2002].

Department of Health and Human Services. 2001. *Medicare Fact Sheet: Providing Coordinated Care to Improve Quality of Care for Chronically Ill Medicare Beneficiaries.* Washington DC: U.S. Department of Health and Human Services.

Finocchio, L., C. Dower, N. Blick, and The Taskforce on Health Care Workforce Regulation. 1998. *Strengthening Consumer Protection: Priorities for Health Care Workforce Regulation.* San Francisco CA: Pew Health Professions Commission.

Health Care Financing Administration. 1998. Medicaid Program; Medicaid Managed Care; Proposed Rule August 20, 2001. 42 CFR §400, 430, et al.

———. 2000. "Quality Improvement System for Managed Care (QISMC) for Organizations Contracting with Medicare or Medicaid. Introduction: Year 2000 Standards and Guidelines. " Online. Available at www.hcfa.gov/quality/3a1.htm [accessed Nov. 9, 2001].

———. 2002. "Medicare Managed Care Manual." Online. Available at www.hcfa.gov/pubforms/86_mmc/mc86toc.htm [accessed Mar. 24, 2002].

Indian Health Service. 2000. "Welcome to the IHPES web site." Online. Available at http://www.ihs.gov/NonMedicalPrograms/IHPES/index.cfm?module=content&option=home [accessed Feb. 15, 2002].

———. 2001a. "Welcome to the Indian Health Service National Diabetes Program." Online. Available at http://www.ihs.gov/medicalprograms/diabetes/ihsndpnewpage.asp [accessed May 9, 2002a].

———. 2001b. "Accreditation Achievement." Online. Available at http://info.ihs.gov/QualityAccount/Quality4.pdf [accessed Mar. 20, 2002b].

Institute of Medicine. 2001a. *Crossing the Quality Chasm: A New Health System for the 21st Century.* Washington DC: National Academy Press.

———. 2001b. An Overview of Major Federal Health Care Quality Programs: A Technical Report for the Institute of Medicine Committee on Enhancing Federal Healthcare Quality Programs. E. K. Swift (ed.). Washington DC: Institute of Medicine.

———. 2001c. *An Overview of Major Federal Health Care Quality Programs: Appendix B.* Washington DC: IOM.

KePRO. 2001. "KePRO: TRICARE." Online. Available at http://www.kepro.org/tricare.htm [accessed Nov. 28, 2001].

Kizer, K. W. 1995. *Vision for Change: A Plan to Restructure the Veterans Health Administration.* Washington DC: U.S. Department of Veterans Affairs.

MedPAC. 1999. Chapter 2: "Influencing Quality in Traditional Medicare". *Report to Congress: Selected Medicare Issues.* Washington DC: MedPAC.

———. 2000. *Report to the Congress: Selected Medicare Issues.* Washington DC: MedPAC.

———. 2001. *Report to the Congress: Medicare Payment for Nursing and Allied Health Education.* Washington DC: MedPAC.

———. 2002. "Report to Congress: Applying Quality Improvement Standards in Medicare." Online. Available at http://www.medpac.gov/publications/congressional_reports/jan2002_QualityImprovement.pdf [accessed Oct. 2, 2002].

National Committee for Quality Assurance. 2002. *HEDIS 2002, Volume 3: Specifications for Survey Measures Information.* Washington DC: NCQA.

NCQA. 2002. "Medicare+Choice (M+C) Deeming Program." Online. Available at http://www.ncqa.org/programs/m+c/m-cmain.htm [accessed May 16, 2002].

Office of Personnel Management. 2002. "Federal Employees Health Benefits Program Home Page." Online. Available at http://www.opm.gov/insure/health/ [accessed Mar. 26, 2002].

Pittman, R., Principal Pharmacy Consultant (Indian Health Service). 26 March 2002. IHS Conditions of Participation, Roles of the Federal and State Governments, and Quality Improvement. Personal communication to Jill Eden.

Rosenfeld, B., T. Dorman, and M. Breslow, et al. 2000. Intensive Care Unit Telemedicine: Alternative Paradigm for Providing Continuous Intensive Care. *Crit Care Med* 28 (12):3925-31.

Sage, W., and L. Aiken. 1997. *Chapter 4: Regulating Interdisciplinary Practice.* In *Regulation of Healthcare Professions.* Chicago, IL: Health Administration Press.

Schuster, M. A., E. A. McGlynn, and R. H. Brook. 1998. How good is the quality of health care in the United States? *Milbank Q* 76 (4):517-63.

Shalala, D. 2000. *Report to Congress: Safeguards for Individuals with Special Health Care Needs Enrolled in Medicaid Managed Care.* Washington DC: Department of Health and Human Services.

TRICARE. 2002. "DoD Centers of Excellence." Online. Available at http://www.tricare.osd.mil/coe/default.cfm [accessed May 6, 2002].

Verdier, J., and R. Dodge. 2002. *Other Data Sources and Uses, Working Paper in the Informed Purchasing Series.* Lawrenceville NJ: Center for Health Care Strategies.

Veterans Administration. 2001. "VHA Handbook 1100.19: Credentialing and Privileging." Online. Available at http://www.va.gov/publ/direc/health/handbook/1100-19HK (3-6-01).pdf [accessed May 8, 2002].

Veterans Health Administration. 2001. Major quality improvement and evaluation programs in the Department of Veterans Affairs: a summary prepared for the Institute of Medicine. Washington DC: U.S. Department of Veterans Affairs.

4

Performance Measures

Summary of Chapter Recommendations

The committee recommends that the federal government accelerate, expand, and coordinate its use of standardized performance measurement and reporting to improve health care quality.

RECOMMENDATION 3: Congress should direct the Secretaries of the Department of Health and Human Services (DHHS), Department of Defense (DOD), and Department of Veterans Affairs (VA) to work together to establish standardized performance measures across the government programs, as well as public reporting requirements for clinicians, institutional providers, and health plans in each program. These requirements should be implemented for all six major government health care programs and should be applied fairly and equitably across various financing and delivery options within those programs. The standardized measurement and reporting activities should replace the many performance measurement activities currently under way in the various government programs.

RECOMMENDATION 4: The Quality Interagency Coordination (QuIC) Task Force should promulgate standardized sets of performance measures for 5 common health conditions in fiscal year (FY) 2003 and another 10 sets in FY 2004.

a.   Each government health care program should pilot test the first 5 sets of measures between FY 2003 and FY 2005 in a limited number

of sites. These pilot tests should include the collection of patient-level data and the public release of comparative performance reports.

   b.   All six government programs should prepare for full implementation of the 15-set performance measurement and reporting system by FY 2008. The government health care programs that provide services through the private sector (i.e., Medicare, Medicaid, the State Children's Health Insurance Program [SCHIP], and portions of DOD TRICARE) should inform participating providers that submission of the audited patient-level data necessary for performance measurement will be required for continued participation in FY 2007. The government health care programs that provide services directly (i.e., the Veterans Health Administration [VHA], the remainder of DOD TRICARE, and the Indian Health Service [IHS]) should begin work immediately to ensure that they have the information technology capabilities to produce the necessary data.

The initial set of measures should focus primarily on validated process-of-care measures. Many process measures, such as those in the Diabetes Quality Improvement Project (DQIP) set, can readily be used for quality measurement without adjusting for patients' demographics or other risk factors. Moreover, compared with outcome measures, many process measures take less time to collect, require smaller samples, and can be collected from data that have already been recorded for other clinical or administrative purposes (Rubin et al., 2001). Process measures can also be easier to benchmark. But the measurement set should not be limited to process measures alone. Over time, incorporating outcome measures and measures of patient perceptions will allow for a richer assessment of the contributions of health care to improved patient and population health status.

The QuIC, an interagency committee with representation from the six major government health care programs, is well positioned to coordinate these activities. QuIC should coordinate its efforts with private-sector groups involved in the promulgation of standardized performance measures, such as the National Quality Forum (NQF), the National Committee for Quality Assurance (NCQA), the Joint Commission on Accreditation of Healthcare Organizations (JCAHO), the Leapfrog Group, and the Foundation for Accountability (FACCT).

The coordinating body should ensure that the design of performance measures and their dissemination reflect the participation of consumers. It should also aim to minimize the number of times providers must report patient-specific performance data. For example, standardized data on patients who are dually eligible for Medicare and Medicaid might be submitted to a clearinghouse, which would then distribute the data to the relevant programs.

In health care, the notion of measuring the performance of clinicians and institutions to improve outcomes is not new. The Pennsylvania Hospital collected diagnosis-specific data on patient outcomes in 1754 (McIntyre et al., 2001). A century later, Florence Nightingale developed a hospital data collection and analysis system that ultimately led to new insights into how sanitary conditions affect hospital morbidity and mortality (Nerenz and Neil, 2001). In 1910, a Massachusetts General Hospital surgeon proposed an "end result" tracking system to determine whether patients had received effective treatments (McIntyre et al., 2001).

The focus in today's health care environment is increasingly on using performance data to measure quality, to demand accountability, and to cultivate an information-rich health care marketplace (American Medical Association, 2001). Performance measurement is commonplace in government health care programs; its application, however, is often uncoordinated and duplicative. As a result, health providers of all types and in all health care settings are increasingly engaged in costly and often redundant measurement and reporting activities to meet the demands of government agencies, accrediting groups, professional associations, and others. In addition, providers serving patients with multiple sources of coverage are further burdened by having to submit the same data to more than one agency in the Centers for Medicare and Medicaid Services (CMS), such as the Medicare and Medicaid programs. With each new measure, there are often different and sometimes conflicting methodologies, data requirements, and terminology (Jencks, 2000; Roper and Cutler, 1998).[1]

This chapter describes some of the leading performance measures used by government health care programs and concludes by setting forth a vision for optimizing the use of performance measurement.

TYPES OF PERFORMANCE MEASURES

Performance measurement in the context of this report is the use of specific quantitative indicators to identify the degree to which providers in the health care system are delivering care that is consistent with standards or acceptable to customers of the delivery system. More than 20

---

[1]The proliferation of measures is well illustrated in a recent review of quality indicators for one diagnosis alone—community-acquired pneumonia (CAP) (Rhew et al., 2001). The authors conducted a systematic search for CAP-specific quality indicators and identified 44 indicators from 10 organizations including CMS, JCAHO, the Agency for Healthcare Research and Quality (AHRQ), and VHA. They concluded that only 16 of the 44 indicators were based on evidence, able to detect "clinically meaningful differences," measurable in a clinical practice setting, or sufficiently precise.

years ago, Donabedian (1980) proposed that quality can be measured by observing its structure, processes, and outcomes. *Structural measures*— such as staffing ratios or the presence of a patient safety committee—refer to organizational characteristics that are thought to create the potential for good quality. They are the basis for most current regulations and are often required by government programs through accreditation, licensure, or certification requirements as a way of ensuring a minimal capacity for quality (as described in Chapter 3).

Process measures quantify the delivery of recommended procedures or services that are correlated with desired outcomes in a specific population group. Process measures can be useful for assessing individual practitioners, as well as for comparing institutional providers, communities, or larger geographic areas (Agency for Healthcare Research and Quality, 2002b). For example, the quality of adult diabetes care is often judged by examining the percent of patients with diabetes who receive recommended services including hemoglobin A1c tests, low-density lipoprotein cholesterol tests, lipid profiles, and retinal exams (Texas Medical Foundation, 2002). The data needed to develop process measures are typically obtained from medical records, claims data, and patient surveys.

Outcome measures are used to capture the effect of an intervention on health status, control of a chronic condition, specific clinical findings, or patients' perceptions of care (Nerenz and Neil, 2001). Two core intermediate outcome measures in adult diabetes care, for example, are the percentage of patients whose most recent hemoglobin A1c level is greater than 9.5 percent and the percentage of patients whose most recent low-density lipoprotein cholesterol level is less than 130 mg/dL. Outcome analysis may require sophisticated statistical techniques, including risk adjustment, to discern the impact of an intervention independent of confounding factors such as comorbidities, socioeconomic characteristics, and local patterns of care (Agency for Healthcare Research Quality, 2002b; Rubin et al., 2001).

Until the QuIC was established in 1998, there was little coordination of government's use of performance measures for quality improvement. The QuIC has initiated projects to address tasks that are key to the use of quality performance measures (Foster, 2002). These include efforts to inventory quality measures; document their uses, strengths, and weaknesses; explore how best to employ risk adjustment methods; encourage all government programs to use the DQIP measures; and identify the most effective ways to communicate with patients about quality, such as establishing a common vocabulary for federal health care agencies (Quality Interagency Coordination, 2002).

COMMONLY USED PERFORMANCE MEASURE SETS

This section describes some of the leading performance measurement sets used by one or more government health care programs (see Table 4-1).

Consumer Assessment of Health Plans

CAHPS is a survey instrument and reporting system developed, with funding and direction from the Agency for Healthcare Research Quality (AHRQ), to help consumers and purchasers choose among health care plans. CAHPS employs primarily outcome measures—specifically consumers' perceptions of their health plan and personal providers—and is used by some state Medicaid agencies, the Medicare program, DOD TRICARE, and public and private employers. NCQA requires managed care plans to field CAHPS and to develop quality improvement projects that address problems identified through CAHPS findings. JCAHO similarly encourages, but does not require, some accredited health care organizations, such as health networks, to employ CAHPS.

CAHPS was originally conceived as a tool for managed care, but more recently has been adapted for fee-for-service (FFS) purposes. There are publicly available algorithms for developing and reporting standardized composite measures of CAHPS results in standardized formats. Comparative analyses of CAHPS outcomes are greatly enhanced through the National CAHPS Benchmarking Database.

The CAHPS initiative is still a work in progress. It remains uncertain whether satisfaction ratings can meaningfully inform quality improvement (Sofaer, 2002). AHRQ has launched the development of a second generation of CAHPS research to evaluate the system's utility for quality improvement and to assess its effectiveness in applied settings. The principal objectives of CAHPS II are to develop innovative reporting formats and to create survey instruments for nursing homes and group practices that can be used by persons with mobility impairments (Agency for Healthcare Research Quality, 2001).

Diabetes Quality Improvement Project

DQIP is an example of a disease-specific performance measurement set. The project was funded by CMS to develop a national consensus with regard to a set of standardized process and outcome measures for performance reporting related to the care of adults with diabetes (see Appendix B) (Texas Medical Foundation, 2002). Although the DQIP measure set has

TABLE 4-1 Selected Performance Measure Sets Used by One or More Government Health Programs

	CAHPS	DQIP	ESRD CPMs	HEDIS	MDS	CMS National Priorities	OASIS
Setting	Health Plans, FFS	Outpatient, hospital	ESRD facilities	Health plans	LTC facilities	Out-patient, hospital	Home Care
Types of Measures	Outcomes	Process	Outcome	Process, outcome, structure	Process, outcome	Process, outcome	Outcome
Medicare	X	X	X	X	X	X	X
Medicaid	X	X		X	X		X
SCHIP	X	X		X			
DOD TRICARE	X	X		X			
VHA	X	X					
IHS		X					

NOTE: CAHPS = Consumer Assessment of Health Plans; CMS = Centers for Medicare and Medicaid Services; DQIP = Diabetes Quality Improvement Project; ESRD CPM = End stage renal disease, clinical performance measure; FFS= Fee for service; HEDIS = Health Plan Employer Data and Information Set; IHS = Indian Health Service; LTC=Long term care; MDS = Minimum data set; OASIS = Outcome Assessment and Information Set; SCHIP = State Children's Health Insurance Program; VHA = Veterans Health Administration.

been evolving,[2] it is being used by all the major government programs, has been incorporated in the Health Plan Employer Data and Information Set (HEDIS) (see below), and is required in CMS managed care contracts (although not in Medicare FFS). DQIP includes abstracting and quality improvement tools as well as a technical assistance hotline.

End Stage Renal Disease Clinical Performance Measures

This set of process and outcome measures is used by CMS to monitor and improve the care provided by dialysis facilities. The measures include indicators of the adequacy of hemodialysis and peritoneal dialysis, vascular access, and anemia management. The public can obtain from the Medicare Website patient survival outcomes as well as other information for any dialysis facility receiving Medicare reimbursement. The ESRD CPMs have been credited for significant improvements in the quality of renal dialysis facilities (Jencks, 2001).

Health Plan Employer Data and Information Set

HEDIS was introduced by NCQA in 1991, and is updated annually to help purchasers and consumers compare the quality of commercial, Medicaid, and Medicare managed care plans. Its measures are used in many government health care programs, particularly in managed care settings. HEDIS incorporates other established standard measure sets, such as CAHPS, DQIP, and the Health Outcomes Survey (HOS). It encompasses the care of common health conditions, including asthma, cancer, depression, diabetes, and heart disease; patients' perceptions of care received; and structural health plan attributes.

Minimum Data Set

The MDS is an 8-page set of core assessment items introduced by CMS in 1990 in all Medicare- and Medicaid-certified nursing homes principally for clinical assessment of nursing home residents. CMS is currently conducting a pilot project that involves regular disclosure of nine risk-adjusted quality measures, derived from the MDS, with the aim of promot-

---

[2]DQIP has been a primary focus of NQF. In May 2002, the NQF Diabetes Measures Review Committee issued for public comment a draft set of diabetes measures drawn from the DQIP measures. The draft set was developed by the National Diabetes Quality Improvement Alliance, a collaboration of the American Medical Association, JCAHO, and NCQA.

ing quality improvement in nursing homes in six states. There are six chronic care measures (e.g., physical restraints, pressure sores, weight loss, infections, residents with pain, and declines in activities of daily living) and three measures of post-acute care quality (e.g., managing delirium, residents with pain, and improvement in walking) (Centers for Medicare and Medicaid Services, 2001c).

MDS and the Outcome Assessment and Information Set (OASIS) (see below) have been criticized for being overly burdensome to providers and for failing to reflect the care patients experience as they move from one health care setting to another, such as the transitions to and from home health care to nursing home and hospital (Institute of Medicine, 2001b).[3] The Medicare, Medicaid, and SCHIP Benefits Improvement and Protection Act of 2000 (Public Law 106-554) mandated that the Secretary of DHHS report to Congress on the development of standard assessment instruments across a wide array of health care settings, including home care and nursing home care.[4] CMS has recently taken steps to shorten the MDS for prospective payment system assessments, effective July 2002 (Centers for Medicare and Medicaid Services, 2002d).

National Priorities Project

This is a CMS quality improvement organization (QIO) project to improve statewide Medicare FFS performance. It uses 22 process measures for three inpatient clinical topics (acute myocardial infarction, heart failure, and stroke) and three outpatient clinical topics (early detection of breast cancer, diabetes management, and pneumonia and influenza immunization).

---

[3]The IOM Committee on Improving Quality in Long-Term Care has recommended that DHHS and others "fund scientifically sound research toward further development of quality assessment instruments that can be used appropriately across the different long-term care settings and different population groups" (Institute of Medicine, 2001b, p. 127).

[4]The report to Congress is due January 1, 2005. It will address issues related to the use of standard instruments for acute care hospitals (in- and out-patient); rehabilitation hospitals (in- and out-patient); skilled nursing facilities; home health agencies; physical, occupational, or speech therapy; ESRD facilities; and partial hospitalization or other mental health services (Johnson, 2001). In 2001, DHHS held a round of initial meetings with more than 200 stakeholders to identify the key issues that should be addressed in the report to Congress. The stakeholders clearly agreed that it would be optimal to use health information standards to collect comparable data (Hines, 2002). Currently, the agency is working to secure funds to extend this effort (Paul, 2002).

Outcome Assessment and Information Set

OASIS is a clinical dataset used by CMS for assessing home care since 1999. CMS requires home care agencies to submit OASIS data for most adult Medicare and Medicaid patients. There have been widespread complaints about the time and expense required to complete the OASIS reporting form. Numerous organizations have called for streamlining of the dataset because of this administrative burden. Critics have maintained that the OASIS reporting requirements are duplicative, that the paperwork involved consumes more nursing time than that devoted to patient care, that associated administrative costs are inadequately reimbursed, and even that OASIS is partly to blame for the critical shortage of qualified home care nurses (American Hospital Association and American Home Care Association, 2001). However, there is evidence that OASIS has been a useful tool in home health quality improvement projects, resulting in measurably better outcomes for patients (Shaughnessy et al., 2002). In June 2002, the DHHS Secretary's Advisory Committee on Regulatory Reform recommended that OASIS be subject to an independent cost–benefit evaluation. The committee also recommended that the reporting form be modernized to, for example, better reflect home health agency operations and current medical practice; to eliminate data elements that are duplicative or not used for payment, quality management, or survey purposes; and to create the option to use one form for all situations of care or changes in status (DHHS Secretary's Advisory Committee on Regulatory Reform, 2002). In response to a request from the Secretary, CMS completed an in-depth review of all OASIS elements and has proposed reducing the burden associated with OASIS by approximately 25 percent. CMS estimates that the proposed changes could be implemented by the end of December 2002. CMS has also convened a technical expert panel and hosted a town hall meeting to assess any additional opportunities for streamlining the OASIS data collection tool (Centers for Medicare and Medicaid Services, 2002e).

OVERVIEW OF CURRENT PERFORMANCE MEASUREMENT ACTIVITIES

Centers for Medicare and Medicaid Services

CMS manages the lion's share of the federal responsibilities for three of the government health care programs addressed in this report—Medicare, Medicaid, and SCHIP. It thereby influences the quality of health care services provided to more than one in four U.S. residents (an estimated 83 million people).

Medicare

Since creating Medicare in 1965, Congress has mandated a series of programs to ensure the quality of care provided to Medicare beneficiaries (Institute of Medicine, 1990). Medicare's approach to improving quality—like that in the private sector—has evolved differently depending on the clinical context and delivery setting (MedPAC, 1999). By statute, Medicare's quality improvement resources must be allocated to its FFS and Medicare+Choice (M+C) programs in proportion to beneficiary participation in the two delivery systems (Health Care Financing Administration, 1999).[5] Nevertheless, CMS relies much more heavily on regulatory requirements to promote quality in Medicare managed care and in long-term care facilities and programs than in Medicare FFS (MedPAC, 2002).[6] In addition, although CMS employs performance measures to stimulate quality improvement across a wide range of clinical settings and delivery systems, it uses those measures in distinctly different ways in managed care and FFS (MedPAC, 2002). For example:

• While M+C plans are held accountable for their performance, FFS contractors are not. As a condition of Medicare participation, M+C plans must implement a quality improvement process and also show evidence of improvement using three sets of measures, including the Medicare versions of HEDIS, CAHPS, and HOS (MedPAC, 2002).[7] In Medicare FFS, participation in quality improvement projects is voluntary (although hospitals and other health care institutions must respond to QIO data requests).

• CMS publicly discloses the quality improvement efforts of individual M+C plans by, for example, annually reporting each plan's HEDIS measures on the CMS Website. Only limited information about relatively small subsets of FFS providers (i.e., dialysis facilities and nursing homes) is publicly reported.

Quality Improvement Organizations

QIOs are Medicare's primary tool for enhancing quality (see Box 4-1). Today's QIOs reflect more than 30 years' evolution in CMS efforts to ad-

---

[5]About 87 percent of Medicare beneficiaries are covered by Medicare fee for service (FFS); 14 percent are enrolled in Medicare+Choice (M+C) and health maintenance organizations (Stuber et al., 2001).

[6]This is due in part to the Balanced Budget Act (BBA) of 1997 (P.L. 105-33), which instructed CMS to regulate quality improvement in M+C plans.

[7]See Chapter 3 for a discussion of Medicare conditions of participation.

BOX 4-1
Quality Improvement Organizations:
Objectives, Staffing, and Financing

There are currently 37 QIOs serving the 50 states, District of Columbia, and U.S. territories. Medicare's QIO program has three basic objectives:

- To improve the quality of care for Medicare beneficiaries by ensuring that it meets professionally recognized standards of health care.
- To protect the integrity of the Medicare Trust Fund by ensuring that Medicare pays only for reasonable and medically necessary services that are provided in the most economical setting.
- To protect beneficiaries by expeditiously addressing beneficiary complaints, provider-issued notices of noncoverage, violations of the Emergency Medical Treatment and Active Labor Act (P.L. 99-272—the anti-dumping statute), payment error prevention, and other mandated responsibilities.

CMS finances QIO projects through competitively awarded contracts that can be renewed every 3 years or canceled and put up for competitive bidding. QIOs are private organizations that vary in their capabilities and the extent to which they do non-Medicare work. They typically employ a multidisciplinary team that includes physicians, nurses, health care quality professionals, epidemiologists, statisticians, and communications experts.
Every QIO contracts with Medicare, but many QIOs also work with state Medicaid programs (about two-thirds conduct quality reviews for state Medicaid agencies) as well as with private employers, skilled nursing facilities, and ESRD facilities.
The Medicare-QIO 3-year contracts detail a complex and extensive set of tasks referred to as the Scope of Work (SOW). During the sixth SOW, covering federal fiscal years 2000-2002, QIOs received about $240 million per year from CMS, approximately one-tenth of 1.0 percent of annual Medicare spending. The seventh SOW was issued while this report was being prepared.

SOURCES: Agency for Healthcare Research and Quality, 2002a; Center for Medicare Education, 2001; Centers for Medicare and Medicaid Services, 2002a; Health Care Financing Administration, 2000; MedPAC, 2002.

dress quality in the Medicare program. As discussed in Chapter 3, these state- or regional-level organizations initially engaged in retrospective review of paper medical records to identify any incidents of poor-quality hospital care and discipline wrongdoers (Institute of Medicine, 1990). Over time, the review organizations became increasingly responsible for protecting the fiscal integrity of the Medicare program and thus were charged with an array of additional responsibilities, such as lowering admission rates, reducing inpatient lengths of stay, providing prior authorizations for some elective procedures, and, just recently, preventing payment errors.

In the 1990s, in response to congressional direction, CMS moved the QIOs towards a more proactive, population- and evidence-based approach to measuring and sometimes disclosing provider and health plan performance. This approach is a clear departure from the past as it deemphasizes punitive actions and instead emphasizes community outreach and collaboration with health plans, providers, and the long-term care industry at the local and regional levels (Center for Medicare Education, 2001).

This shift became evident in the fifth SOW (1997–1999) and sixth SOW (2000–2002) and is further emphasized in the seventh SOW (2003–2005) (Centers for Medicare and Medicaid Services, 2001e). The heart of the sixth SOW was the National Priorities project to improve statewide Medicare FFS performance. As noted earlier, this effort involves the use of the same 22 clinical performance measures nationwide for three inpatient clinical topics (acute myocardial infarction [AMI], heart failure, and stroke) and three outpatient clinical topics (early detection of breast cancer, diabetes management, and pneumonia and influenza immunization). Each clinical topic is supported by a Medicare-designated QIO that provides technical support on that topic to QIOs nationwide (see Table 4-2).

The QIOs use the 22 performance measures to determine their state's or region's baseline performance for each clinical topic, work with local providers to make improvements, and report state-level results to CMS. They typically offer local providers clinical documentation supporting the performance indicators, feedback data on actual performance, and technical advice on alternatives for improving systems, and also convene meetings to promote collaboration among local stakeholders (Jencks, 2002). Medicare does not require individual clinicians to work with the QIOs on any specific improvement project (MedPAC, 2002). Thus, QIOs must find ways to persuade local providers to collaborate with them if they are to achieve state-level improvements in the performance measures.

The sixth SOW also required every QIO to offer technical assistance to all the M+C plans in its state (Health Care Financing Administration,

TABLE 4-2 National Medicare QIO Projects in the 6th SOW

Clinical Topic (Lead QIO)	Clinical Setting	Performance Measures (% of beneficiaries receiving unless otherwise indicated)	Data Sources
Acute Myocardial Infarction (AMI) (Qualidigm, <CTMedicare.org/ ami_caspro>)	Hospitals	Early administration of aspirin after arrival at hospital	Hospital medical records for
		Early administration of beta blocker after arrival at hospital	AMI patients
		Time to initiation of reperfusion therapy	
		Aspirin at discharge	
		Beta blocker at discharge	
		Angiotensin-converting enzyme (ACE) inhibitor at discharge for systolic dysfunction	
		Smoking cessation counseling during hospitalization	
Breast Cancer Early Detection (Virginia Health Quality Center, <vhqc.org>)	Doctors' offices, outpatient settings	Biennial mammogram	Medicare claims for all female beneficiaries
Diabetes (Texas Medical Foundation, <dqip.org and tmf.org>)	Doctors' offices, outpatient settings	Biennial retinal exam by an eye professional	Medicare claims for all diabetic beneficiaries
		Annual hemoglobin A1c (HbA1c) testing	
		Biennial lipid profile	
Heart failure (Colorado Foundation for Medical Care, <national heartfailure.org>)	Hospitals	Appropriate use/nonuse of ACE inhibitors at discharge (excluding discharges on Angiotension-II Receptor Blocker)	Hospital medical records for heart failure patients

continued

TABLE 4-2 Continued

Clinical Topic (Lead QIO)	Clinical Setting	Performance Measures (% of beneficiaries receiving unless otherwise indicated)	Data Sources
Pneumonia and influenza (Oklahoma Foundation for Medical Quality, <nationalpneumonia.org and ofmq.com>)	Doctors' offices, outpatient settings	State influenza vaccination rate	Centers for Disease Control and Prevention's Behavioral Risk Factor Surveillance System Data; hospital medical records for pneumonia patients
		State pneumococcal vaccination rate	
		Influenza vaccination or screening	
		Pneumococcal vaccination or screening	
		Blood culture before antibiotics are administered	
		Administration of antibiotics consistent with current recommendations	
		Initial antibiotic dose within 8 hours of hospital arrival	
Stroke (Iowa Foundation for Medical Quality <ifmc.org>)	Hospitals	Discharged on antithrombotic (acute stroke or transient ischemic attack [TIA])	Hospital medical records for stroke, TIA, and chronic atrial fibrillation patients
		Discharged on warfarin (atrial fibrillation)	
		Avoidance of sublingual nifedipine (acute stroke)	

SOURCE: Adapted from Centers for Medicare and Medicaid Services, 2002b.

1999).[8] Much of this assistance is focused on helping the plans to interpret their HEDIS, CAHPS, and HOS results, to identify opportunities for improving care, and to develop and evaluate measurable interventions.[9] QIOs are also required to work with ESRD facilities, home-health agen-

---

[8]The BBA established Part C of Medicare (i.e., the M+C program), which became effective in January 2000.
[9]HEDIS technical specifications are updated annually.

cies, and long-term care facilities (Centers for Medicare and Medicaid Services, 2002a).

ORYX

As described in the previous chapter, Medicare and most other government programs rely on JCAHO accreditation to help ensure a minimal level of health care quality. Performance measurement has become an integral component of JCAHO accreditation. JCAHO's ORYX initiative requires accredited hospitals, long-term care facilities, home care providers, and behavioral care organizations to routinely submit patient-level data for performance measurement and to regularly demonstrate how they use performance measures to monitor and improve the quality of their services (see Box 4-2).

End Stage Renal Disease

The legislation that created the ESRD program in 1972 (Section 2991, Public Law 92-603), established ESRD Network Coordinating Councils as the official liaisons between the nation's ESRD providers and the federal government (Forum of End Stage Renal Disease Networks, 2002). The 19 ESRD networks are CMS' principal instruments for encouraging quality improvements in ESRD services. The networks' scope of work is determined by competitively awarded contracts with CMS that delineate specific quality improvement activities as well as numerous other tasks. The quality improvement efforts are based on the premise that ESRD networks "can do more to improve the quality and cost effectiveness of care by bringing typical care into line with the best practices rather than by inspecting individual cases to identify erred treatment" (Centers for Medicare and Medicaid Services, 2001a, p.1)

Routine collection and analysis of clinical performance measures are a principal initiative of the program. The ESRD clinical performance measures are calculated from annual national random samples of adult dialysis patients. Each year, ESRD facilities with one or more patients in the sample must submit an array of patient-specific data to their respective ESRD network. According to their trade association, the networks maintain the world's largest, comprehensive disease-specific registry. It includes Medicare beneficiaries, non-Medicare patients, Medicare secondary patients, and Veterans Health Administration (VHA) patients (Forum of End Stage Renal Disease Networks, 2002).

CMS maintains a Dialysis Facility Compare Website where members of the public can view selected clinical performance measures, such as adequacy of dialysis and patient survival, for the approved Medicare

BOX 4-2
ORYX: JCAHO's Performance Measurement Initiative

Although JCAHO is a private accreditation group, it has a significant impact on almost all health care services provided by government health care programs. JCAHO has statutory authority under Medicare and Medicaid to certify hospitals, ambulatory surgical centers, clinical laboratories, home health agencies, and hospices as being in compliance with the government's minimum standards of participation. JCAHO accreditation is also an important component of the VHA, TRICARE, and IHS health care programs.

ORYX is an evolving initiative, first introduced in February 1997, to support and foster quality improvement in JCAHO-accredited organizations. ORYX integrates outcome and other performance measurement data into the survey and accreditation process for hospitals, long-term care facilities, home care, and behavioral health organizations.

Under the current ORYX program, JCAHO has designated ORYX-certified performance measurement vendors for accredited hospitals, long-term care facilities, home care, and behavioral health organizations. JCAHO requires its accredited organizations to contract with one of the certified vendors. Accredited health care organizations select their performance measures and submit the necessary patient-level data to the vendors who in turn aggregate and report the performance data to JCAHO. JCAHO staff analyze the data, using control and comparison charts, to identify performance trends and patterns. JCAHO surveyors use these analyses to focus their on-site surveys. The accredited applicants must demonstrate that they use the measures to improve their performance.

Hospitals must select performance measures from two of four core measurement areas: acute myocardial infarction, heart failure, community-acquired pneumonia, and pregnancy and related conditions. Since July 1, 2002, hospitals have been collecting performance data for all patient discharges, and they will begin transmitting data to JCAHO via a certified vendor no later than January 31, 2003. Subsequently, quarterly transmissions must be made no later than 4 months after the close of a calendar quarter. Aggregate data from all JCAHO-accredited hospitals will comprise the comparison group for JCAHO's assessment of how each accredited organization uses the performance measurement data for quality improvement.

JCAHO has not yet identified core measures for non-hospital organizations. Until this is done, non-hospital entities may choose their own measures from those measures offered by certified performance measurement vendors.

SOURCE: Joint Commission on Accreditation of Healthcare Organizations, 2002.

ESRD facilities in their own geographic area (Medicare, 2002). There has been an apparent steady improvement in a number of the measures (Centers for Medicare and Medicaid Services, 2001e; Jencks, 2001). For example, during the period 1993–1999, the proportion of adult dialysis patients receiving inadequate dialysis treatment declined from 57 to 20 percent. At the same time, the proportion of adult dialysis patients with anemia dropped from 57 to 32 percent.

Home Health Care

Since 1999, CMS has used OASIS for its oversight of home health agencies participating in the Medicare and Medicaid programs. All Medicare-certified home care agencies must collect, computerize, and electronically transmit OASIS data at regular intervals to a CMS-approved central source for all their adult Medicare or Medicaid patients receiving personal care or health services (42 Code of Federal Regulations Part 484). CMS's seventh SOW for QIOs directs them to help home health agencies develop quality improvement projects using OASIS-based performance measures (Centers for Medicare and Medicaid Services, 2002c). Eventually, CMS plans to generate outcome reports for all certified home care agencies.

Skilled Nursing Care

All certified long-term care facilities, such as nursing homes and skilled nursing facilities, must transmit to their state an MDS drawn from residents' medical records; in turn, the states submit the data to CMS (Centers for Medicare and Medicaid Services, 2001b). Members of the public can now consult the CMS website to view several nursing home quality measures, such as the percent of residents with pressure sores, the percent with urinary incontinence, and summary results from state nursing home inspections for facilities in their own geographic area and throughout the nation (Centers for Medicare and Medicaid Services, 2001c).

In April 2002, CMS initiated a six-state pilot to identify, collect, and publish nursing home quality information in Colorado, Florida, Maryland, Ohio, Rhode Island, and Washington. The project, which draws from CMS' collaboration with the NQF to identify nine risk-adjusted quality measures for use by beneficiaries (Centers for Medicare and Medicaid Services, 2002f), uses measures which target the quality of both chronic care and post-acute care.

Medicaid

Since the Medicaid program was created by Congress in 1965, states have had great flexibility in how they manage their Medicaid programs. The same is also generally true of how states conduct Medicaid quality assurance and improvement activities. Government rules grant states wide latitude in establishing their own goals for Medicaid quality and in choosing the methods they use to achieve these goals. For example, CMS requires states to collect Medicaid encounter data, but the states are free to determine many of the specific features of the data, including the data elements themselves, reporting frequency, and level of aggregation (Matthews, 2000). As a consequence, state-to-state comparisons of Medicaid quality are largely infeasible.

Performance measures have become a popular state tool for assessing and promoting quality improvement in Medicaid managed care, but there are few useful quality performance measures for Medicaid FFS health care. Most states use a combination of publicly available measures and state-developed measures for Medicaid managed care (Kaye, 2001). In 2000, Medicaid HEDIS and Medicaid CAHPS were the most common national measure sets used by the states. However, states usually modify the specifications to tailor data collection to their own specific program needs (French and Miele, 2001). Many states have developed consumer report cards drawing from HEDIS, CAHPS, and other performance measures (Verdier and Dodge, 2002). Many states have also implemented provider incentive programs that employ performance indicators (Dyer et al., 2002).

Despite the variation in states' HEDIS data specifications, the NCQA and the American Public Human Services Association have established a national database of Medicaid HEDIS statistics. In 2001, the database incorporated 168 individual Medicaid managed care plan HEDIS submissions (for 29 plans the data were unaudited). NCQA reports that although there were across-the-board improvements in commercial plans' HEDIS performance, from 1998 to 2000, Medicaid performance was mixed (French and Miele, 2001).

There may be greater uniformity in performance data for Medicaid managed care once CMS implements related rules under the Balanced Budget Act of 1997, which directed CMS to develop specific protocols to guide the states' conduct of external quality review of Medicaid managed care plans. In their current form, the protocols assume that states will continue to have flexibility in developing performance measures because they will be required to conduct their performance reviews only in a manner *consistent with* but not necessarily identical to the protocols (Centers for Medicare and Medicaid Services, 2001d).[10] States will be free to specify

---

[10]The draft protocols were still out for public comment while this report was being prepared.

their performance measures, the specifications to be followed in calculating the measures, and the method and timing that health plans must use for reporting.[11]

State Children's Health Insurance Program

Congress established the SCHIP program in 1997 for low-income uninsured children. As of 2002, most states had operated their programs for only 3 or 4 years. As a consequence, both the federal and state focus for SCHIP has been on enrolling eligible children and making the program operational. More recently, attention has turned to assessing the program's efforts (Henneberry, 2001).

SCHIP regulations require states to establish performance goals and performance measures, including a written assurance that the state will collect and maintain data and furnish reports to the Health and Human Services Secretary. Managed care is the dominant delivery system used by SCHIP programs, and the regulations grant CMS the authority to mandate standardized performance measures for managed care plans serving SCHIP enrollees (but not for FFS providers). No specific performance measures or goals are required.

Many states require managed care plans that serve SCHIP enrollees to report HEDIS measures (Henneberry, 2001). However, surveys of SCHIP programs indicate that the programs often modify HEDIS to tailor data collection to their specific program needs thus making state-to-state comparisons problematic (French and Miele, 2001). Some states are also adapting HEDIS for FFS and primary care case management. Other states have developed their own performance measures. Wisconsin, for example, is developing a new performance measurement system, the "Medicaid Encounter Data Driven Improvement Core-Measure Set," drawing directly from monthly HMO encounter data (Henneberry, 2001).

CMS and AHRQ are currently collaborating on a Performance Measurement Partnership Project with state Medicaid and SCHIP programs to determine the feasibility of implementing a core set of standardized performance measures, such as HEDIS or CAHPS, for managed care in Medicaid and SCHIP. One aim of the project is to motivate benchmarking and state creativity in using performance measures (Block, 2002).

---

[11]States may choose to develop their own measures or use standardized measures from HEDIS, FACCT, AHRQ's CONQUEST database, or the measures recommended in *A Guide for States to Assist in the Collection and Analysis of Medicaid Managed Care* (MEDSTAT, 1998).

DOD TRICARE

DOD TRICARE is in the midst of an ambitious effort to reengineer the military health system (MHS) (Milbank Memorial Fund, 2001). In December 2001, TRICARE Management Activity (TMA), the DOD-level administrator of the MHS, released the *Population Health Improvement Plan (PHI) and Guide*, a detailed blueprint for making "population health improvement a reality in the DOD" (DOD TRICARE Management Activity, 2001, p. i). In earlier research that contributed to the guide's development, TMA had concluded that its system was "replete with metrics covering a wide range of uncoordinated indicators of varying usefulness" and "disparate performance measurement systems" (TRICARE, 1999b, p. 26). The PHI Guide directly addresses this concern and calls for an "enterprise-wide core set of standardized performance measures" to drive improvements in clinical services (DOD TRICARE Management Activity, 2001, p. 67). One of the first steps will be to integrate measure sets that are already collected for mandatory quality assurance programs such as HEDIS and ORYX.

Today's TRICARE Website reports numerous performance measurement activities—analyses of HEDIS data used to focus quality improvement efforts related to diabetes, asthma, breast cancer screening, and cervical cancer screening; "report cards" drawn from an array of beneficiary surveys; digests of performance measures called TRICARE Operational Performance Statements (TOPS); and others.

One survey, the *Health Care Survey of DOD Beneficiaries*, is an adapted CAHPS instrument used by TRICARE to monitor consumer satisfaction with and perceptions of the quality of MHS hospitals, clinics, and clinical staff (including how the MHS compares with the care received by the privately insured population) (TRICARE, 1999a).[12] The survey responses are aggregated into composite performance measures using CAHPS algorithms. The resulting measures are benchmarked against the National CAHPS Benchmarking Database and the findings are released in Web-based interactive report cards.

TOPS is a quarterly digest that disseminates routine analyses of the MHS. Included are performance measures such as beneficiary grievance rates, preventable admission rates for active-duty personnel (e.g., for angina or chronic obstructive pulmonary disease), preventable admission rates for non–active duty managed care enrollees (e.g., for asthma or congestive heart failure), access to care, and patient satisfaction.

---

[12]The Health Care Survey of DOD Beneficiaries was mandated by the National Defense Authorization Act for fiscal year 1993 (P.L. 102-484).

Veterans Health Administration

VHA's integrated health information system, including its framework for using performance measures to improve quality, is considered one of the best in the nation. VHA uses performance measures along a number of dimensions—patient satisfaction, functional outcomes, personal health practices, and clinical measures—to drive quality improvement in a wide range of clinical disciplines and across ambulatory, hospital, and long-term care settings (Jones and VHA, 2002; Nerenz and Neil, 2001).

One of the most highly regarded VHA initiatives employing performance measures is the National Surgical Quality Improvement Program (NSQIP). NSQIP was implemented to develop comparative risk-adjusted information on surgical outcomes in the VHA's many medical centers (Daley, 1998). The initiative's key components are periodic performance measurement and feedback, along with comparative, site-specific, and outcome-based annual reports; self-assessment tools; structured site visits; and dissemination of best practices. From 1991, when NSQIP data were first collected, through 2000, the impact on the outcomes of major surgeries at VHA hospitals was dramatic: 30-day postoperative mortality decreased by 27 percent and 30-day morbidity by 45 percent (Shukri et al., 2002).

Many other performance measures are in use, including, for example, several evidence-based quality indices developed by VHA researchers to improve preventive, chronic, and palliative services and commercially available measurement sets such as HEDIS and CAHPS. The Chronic Disease Care Index targets the five most common conditions treated at VHA hospitals: ischemic heart disease, hypertension, chronic obstructive pulmonary disease, diabetes mellitus, and obesity. HEDIS measures have been used to assess diabetes care, heart attack treatment, ambulatory follow-up after inpatient mental health stays, and cervical cancer screening (Jones et al., 2000; Mencke et al., 2000).

Indian Health Service

IHS has developed a performance evaluation system to meet the performance measurement requirements of JCAHO's ORYX initiative and to comply with the Government Performance and Results Act (Indian Health Service, 2000). The majority of IHS facilities are JCAHO-accredited and thus are required to regularly submit and use performance measures for quality improvement. The performance evaluation system uses quality indicators that have been specifically tailored to Indian health care populations and focus on 12 priority health problems: diabetes, obesity, cancer, heart disease, alcohol and substance abuse, family abuse and violence, injuries, dental disease, poor living environment, mental health, tobacco use, and maternal and child health (Indian Health Service, 2002).

OPTIMIZING THE GOVERNMENT'S USE OF PERFORMANCE MEASURES

In its recent comprehensive assessment of how to advance the quality of the MHS, DOD/TMA concluded that a conceptual framework is key for "improving the health of populations" and for guiding the "specific actions and tools that will help to build healthy communities" (DOD TRICARE Management Activity, 2001, p. v). The committee agrees and believes this to be true for all government health care performance measurement efforts. The committee believes further that a conceptual framework for performance measurement should build on efforts already under way.

To achieve the continuity required to formulate a conceptual framework for performance measurement, the committee encouraged adoption of the taxonomy developed by the Institute of Medicine's earlier Committee on the Quality of Health Care in America. That committee identified six dimensions or attributes of quality that should shape government's use of performance measures (see Box 4-3). These six attributes have al-

---

BOX 4-3
Six Attributes of Quality

- *Safe*—avoiding injuries to patients from the care that is intended to help them.
- *Effective*—providing services based on scientific knowledge to all who could benefit and refraining from providing services to those not likely to benefit (avoiding underuse and overuse).
- *Patient-centered*—providing care that is respectful of and responsive to individual patient preferences, needs, and values and ensuring that patient values guide all clinical decisions.
- *Timely*—reducing waits and sometimes harmful delays for both those who receive and those who give care.
- *Efficient*—avoiding waste, in particular waste of equipment, supplies, ideas, and energy.
- *Equitable*—providing care that does not vary in quality because of personal characteristics such as gender, ethnicity, geographic location, and socioeconomic status.

SOURCE: Institute of Medicine, 2001a.

ready been adopted by DHHS as a conceptual framework for the National Health Care Quality Report. They have also been endorsed in whole or in part by various private-sector groups including the Leapfrog Group and NQF. In addition, another IOM committee has identified a list of 20 priority areas for health system improvement, and these represent excellent candidates for the development of standardized performance measures (Institute of Medicine, 2002). Most of the government programs have identified leading chronic conditions and health concerns for their populations, and there is much overlap in all of these lists.

NEED TO STANDARDIZE QUALITY PERFORMANCE MEASURES

Government health care programs reflect a growing recognition that measuring quality and using quality performance measures to improve health care is central to the federal government's roles of regulator, purchaser, and provider of health care for almost half the U.S. population. Yet too many resources are spent on health care measures that are either duplicative or ineffective, and little comparative quality information is made available in the public domain for use by beneficiaries, health professionals, or other stakeholders. Furthermore, potential users of the available measures are often hindered by the lack of reporting standards, conflicting methodologies, and inconsistent terminology (Eddy, 1998; Rhew et al., 2001). Standardizing measures can lessen the confusion. In addition to addressing these problems, the committee believes standardized performance measures could drive quality improvement in numerous other ways:

- By drawing attention to best practices and encouraging providers to adopt them.
- By facilitating comparisons of accountable entities, such as hospitals, health plans, long-term care facilities, and, potentially, physicians' practices.
- By enabling the development of national benchmarks and helping to identify regional differences.
- By supporting efforts to sensibly reward quality through either payment or other means.
- By expanding the research community's capacity to identify the factors that drive or diminish health care quality.
- By helping to make the link between accountable entities and patient outcomes.
- By providing the clinical data needed to formulate workable risk adjustment techniques.
- By providing the necessary data to identify providers who demon-

strate consistently substandard care and developing strategies for improvement or narrowing of their scope of practice.

Performance measurement is not a perfect solution. There are problems and pitfalls with this approach that must be addressed and guarded against. Any performance measurement approach will focus on only a limited number of areas, and there is the risk that too little attention will be paid to clinical areas that are not the focus of measurement activity. There are numerous methodologic challenges, such as capturing rare events and adjusting for differences in risk or severity of illness (Eddy, 1998). In the case of outcome measures, it must be recognized that almost all outcomes are probabilistic (i.e., doing the right things does not guarantee good outcomes, and good outcomes sometimes occur even when the right things were not done), and there are also many factors outside the control of the health system determining outcomes (Eddy, 1998). There must also be ways to identify and deal with missing or incorrect data (McGlynn and Adams, 2001).

While not a perfect solution, the committee believes that the potential benefits of performance measurement and reporting are sizable and that the federal government should act expeditiously to promulgate a standardized measurement set and to implement this set within each of the government programs. At the same time, efforts must be made to address operational and methodologic challenges and to mitigate any unintended adverse consequences.

Implications for Current Activities

Adoption of a central focus on performance measurement and reporting will have significant implications for the way in which the government conducts its quality enhancement activities. In today's environment of scarce resources and rising health care costs, it will be imperative for each government health care program to assess carefully how best to realize its objectives. Standardized quality measurement and reporting must not be pursued as an *additional* government requirement, but rather as a *replacement* for current quality measurement activities. Moreover, whenever possible, providers should not be burdened with reporting the same patient-specific performance data more than once to the same government agency.

There should be a designated government entity responsible for coordinating the government's performance measurement activities. QuIC has made a strong start in the right direction by convening representatives from the six major government health care programs and initiating various collaborative projects based on voluntary participation, but it lacks a clear mandate. Congress should grant the statutory authority and provide adequate funding to either QuIC or another existing entity to coordinate and standardize the government's performance measurement activities. This entity should establish strong working relationships with various private-sector groups, including NQF, NCQA, JCAHO, the Leapfrog Group, and FACCT to optimize future public–private collaboration and provide structured mechanisms for consumer input.

It should be noted that the committee considered and rejected the option of establishing a new oversight authority. It concluded that the existing infrastructure, if applied more rigorously and with adequate resources, has the potential to accomplish the objectives laid out in this report. The costs and organizational challenges of forming a new agency were viewed as substantial, creating the potential for delay in implementation of the substantive activities.

The QuIC should move aggressively to establish an initial set of standardized measures. As noted previously, a wealth of measures already exists. In very few instances will it be necessary to develop measures from scratch. There are some measure sets, for example, DQIP, that are already being used by several or most of the government programs. By starting with this "low hanging fruit," it should be possible to identify measure sets for 5 conditions almost immediately, thus allowing the pilot testing process to begin in fiscal year 2003. The remaining 10 sets can then be designated in fiscal year 2004. By moving expeditiously to designating all 15 sets of measures within the first 18 months to 2 years, the federal government will be providing important information to providers regarding the necessary capabilities and specifications for their information systems.

CMS has historically allocated most of Medicare's quality improvement budget to its QIO contracts. The committee strongly recommends the use of standardized measures derived from computerized data and public reporting of comparative quality information. It will be important for CMS to reexamine how best to use the QIOs to enhance quality within this context. For example, should QIOs play a role in the release of public-domain comparative quality reports? Would substantial quality improvements in Medicare be achieved more readily with fewer QIO-like entities operating on a national or larger regional scale?

States will also need to relinquish some flexibility in promulgating state-specific performance measures for Medicaid and SCHIP programs. State representatives should be active participants in the QuIC, thus having input into the process of establishing the standardized measure sets. But individual states would be required to apply within their Medicaid and SCHIP programs the standardized measures applicable to the populations served. States would still retain a good deal of flexibility in how they use their regulatory and purchasing powers to act on the performance information provided through standardized reporting mechanisms.

In summary, the six major government health care programs should commit to the use of common sets of standardized performance measures. The current administrative burden on the providers that constitute the foundation of government health care services is unacceptable. The committee believes that standardized metrics and reporting formats would not only aid in alleviating this burden, but also help ensure meaningful gains in the quality of health care.

Finally, effective performance measurement demands real time access to sufficient clinical detail and accurate data (Schneider et al., 1999). By the time retrospective performance measures reach decision makers, it is too late for them to be useful. The current health information environment is far too fragmented, technologically primitive, and overly dependent on paper medical records. The nation's need for a functional health care information system is examined in the next chapter.

REFERENCES

Agency for Healthcare Research Quality. 2001. "*AHRQ Seeks Applications for Second Phase of CAHPS®*. Media Advisory." Online. Available at http://www.ahrq.gov/news/press/pr2001/cahps2pr.htm [accessed July 10, 2002].

———. 2002a. "Fact Sheet: Medicare QIOs: Improving Patient Safety and Quality of Care for Seniors; A National Network of Quality Improvement Experts: Major Medicare QIO Efforts." Online. Available at http://www. ahqa.org/pub/media/159_766_2687.cfm [accessed May 13, 2002].

———. 2002b. "Child Health Tool Box: Measuring Performance in Child Health Programs. Understanding Performance Measurement." Online. Available at http://www.ahrq.gov/chtoolbx/understn.htm [accessed July 10, 2002].

American Hospital Association, and American Home Care Association. 2001. Letter to T. Scully, CMS Administrator (Subject: Oasis).

American Medical Association, Joint Commission on Accreditation of Healthcare Organizations and National Committee for Quality Assurance. 2001. "Principles for Performance Measurement in Health Care. A Consensus Statement." Online. Available at http://www.ncqa.org/communications/news/prinpls.htm [accessed May 29, 2002].

Block, R. (CMS). 16 May 2002. Personal communication to Jill Eden.

Center for Medicare Education. 2001. "The Role of PROs, Issue Brief, V2 (2)." Online. Available at http://www.medicareed.org/pdfs/papers53.pdf [accessed May 13, 2002].

Centers for Medicare and Medicaid Services. 2001a. "End Stage Renal Disease (ESRD) Network Organizations." Online. Available at http://www.hcfa.gov/quality/5d.htm [accessed Feb. 8, 2002a].

———. 2001b. "MDS Quality Indicator and Frequencies Reports." Online. Available at http://hcfa.gov/projects/mdsreports/default.asp [accessed June 17, 2002b].

———. 2001c. "Nursing Home Compare—Home." Online. Available at http://www.medicare.gov/NHCompare/home.asp [accessed May 6, 2002c].

———. 2001d. "Protocols for External Quality Review of Medicaid Managed Care Organizations and Prepaid Health Plans." Online. Available at http://www.hcfa.gov/Medicaid/mceqrhmp.htm [accessed May 15, 2002d].

————. 2001e. "Quality of Care: National Projects, ESRD Clinical Performance Measures Project (2000 Annual Report)." Online. Available at hcfa.gov/quality/3m8.htm [accessed Jan. 9, 2002e].

————. 2002a. "Quality Improvement Organizations Statement of Work." Online. Available at www.hcfa.gov/qio/2.asp [accessed Apr. 22, 2002a].

————. 2002b. "Quality Indicators." Online. Available at http://www.cms.hhs.gov/qio/1a1-d.asp [accessed June 14, 2002b].

————. 2002c. "Statement of Work, QIOs: 7th Round February 2002 Version." Online. Available at http://www.hcfa.gov/qio/2b.pdf [accessed May 13, 2002c].

————, CMS Office of Public Affairs. 2002d. "Medicare Streamlines Paperwork Requirements for Nursing Homes to Allow Nurses, Other Caregivers to Spend More Time With Patients." Online. Available at www.CMS.hhs.gov/media/press/release.asp?counter=462. [accessed July 10, 2002d].

————. 2002e. "Medicare Program; Town Hall Meeting on the Outcome Assessment Information Set (OASIS)." Online [accessed Aug. 12, 2002e].

————. "Nursing Home Quality Initiative." Online [accessed Aug. 12, 2002f].

Daley, J. 1998. About the National VA Surgical Quality Improvement Program. *The Forum, VA Office of Research & Develoment.*

DHHS Secretary's Advisory Committee on Regulatory Reform. 2002. Regional Hearing #5 Meeting Minutes/Summary.

DOD TRICARE Management Activity. 2001. "Population Health Improvement Plan Guide." Online. Available at http://www.tricare.osd.mil/mhsophsc/DoD_PHI_Plan_Guide.html [accessed May 15, 2002].

Donabedian, A. 1980. The definition of quality and approaches to its assessment. In *Explorations in Quality Assessment and Monitoring.* Vol. I. Ann Arbor MI: Health Administration Press.

Dyer, M., M. Bailit, and C. Kokenyesi. 2002. *Are Incentives Effective in Improving the Performance of Managed Care Plans, Working Paper in the Informed Purchasing Series.* Lawrenceville NJ: Center for Health Care Strategies.

Eddy, D. M. 1998. Performance measurement: problems and solutions. *Health Aff (Millwood)* 17 (4):7-25 .

Forum of End Stage Renal Disease Networks. 2002. "What Are the ESRD Networks?" Online. Available at http://www.esrdnetworks.org/networks_defined.htm [accessed Apr. 30, 2002].

Foster, N. (QuIC). 18 April 2002. Personal communication to Jill Eden.

French, J. B., and A. Miele. "Evaluation of HEDIS in Medicaid and SCHIP." Online. Available at http://www.ncqa.org/Programs/QSG/EvaluationofHEDISinMedicaidand SCHIP.pdf [accessed Dec. 2001].

Health Care Financing Administration. 1999. "QIO SOWs: Request for Proposal, Sixth Round." Online. Available at http://www.hcfa.gov/qio/2a.pdf [accessed May 13, 2002].

————. 2000. "National Projects Reports: Medicare Priorities." Online. Available at http://www.hcfa.gov/quality/3k.htm#priority [accessed May 13, 2002].

Henneberry, J. 2001. *State efforts to evaluate the progress and success of SCHIP (Issue Brief).* NGA Center for Best Practices.

Hines, L. (DHHS). 8 August 2002. BIPA info. Personal communication to Jill Eden.

Indian Health Service. 2000. "Indian Health Performance Evaluation System (PES)." Online. Available at http://www.ihs.gov/NonMedicalPrograms/IHPES/index.cfm?module=content&option=pes [accessed June 15, 2001].

————. "IHS FY 1999 Performance Plan." Online. Available at http://www.ihs.gov/PublicInfo/Publications/Perfplan2-1-99.asp [accessed Jan. 14, 2002].

Institute of Medicine. 1990. *Medicare: a Strategy for Quality Assurance.* Washington DC: National Academy Press.

———. 2001a. *Crossing the Quality Chasm: A New Health System for the 21st Century.* Washington DC: National Academy Press.

———. 2001b. *Improving the Quality of Long-Term Care.* Washington DC: National Academy Press.

———. 2002. *Priority Areas for National Action: Transforming Health Care Quality.* Washington DC: National Academy Press.

Jencks, S. F. 2000. Clinical performance measurement—a hard sell. *JAMA* 283 (15):2015-6.

Jencks, S. F. 2001. "Oct. workshop: Protecting and Improving Safety and Quality for Medicare-HCQIP." (PP slides).

Jencks, S. F. (Quality Improvement Group, Office of Clinical Standards and Quality, Centers for Medicare & Medicaid Services). 6 August 2002. Re: study period. Personal communication to Jill Eden.

Johnson, D. 2001. *HCFA Legislative Summary: Letter to All Interested Parties.* Washington DC: CMS.

Joint Commission on Accreditation of Healthcare Organizations. 2002. "ORYX: The Next Evolution in Accreditation; Questions and Answers about the Joint Commission's Planned Integration of Performance Measures into the Accreditation Process." Online. Available at http://www.jcaho.org/perfmeas/oryx_qa.html [accessed May 13, 2002].

Jones, D., A. Hendricks, C. Comstock, A. Rosen, B. H. Chang, J. Rothendler, C. Hankin, and M. Prashker. 2000. Eye examinations for VA patients with diabetes: standardizing performance measures. *Int J Qual Health Care* 12 (2):97-104.

Jones, E., and VHA. 2002. "Quality Resources Newsletter; Three Interlinked Services Available in 2002." Online. Available at http://www.oqp.med.va.gov/newsletter/newsletter.asp [accessed May 15, 2002].

Kaye, N. 2001. *Medicaid Managed Care: A Guide for States. Prepared for the Henry J. Kaiser Family Foundation, the Health Resources and Services Administration, the David and Lucile Packard Foundation, and the Congressional Research Service.* Portland ME: National Academy for State Health Policy.

Matthews, T. L. 2000. *Measuring the Quality of Medicaid Managed Care: An Introduction to State Efforts.* Lexington KY: Council Of State Governments.

McGlynn, E., and J. Adams. 2001. Public release of information on quality. Pp. 183-202. In *Changing the U.S. Health Care System: Key Issues in Health Services Policy and Management.* 2nd edition. R. Andersen, T. Rice, and G. Kominksi, eds. Jossey-Bass, Inc.

McIntyre, D., L. Rogers, and E. J. Heier. 2001. Overview, history and objectives of performance measurement. *Health Care Financ Rev* 22 (3):7-21.

Medicare. 2002. "Medicare.gov - Dialysis Facility Compare Home." Online. Available at http://www.medicare.gov/dialysis/home.asp [accessed May 13, 2002].

MedPAC. 1999. Chapter 2: "Influencing Quality in Traditional Medicare." *Report to Congress: Selected Medicare Issues.* Washington DC: MedPAC.

———. 2002. "Report to Congress: Applying Quality Improvement Standards in Medicare." Online. Available at http://www.medpac.gov/publications/congressional_reports/jan2002_QualityImprovement.pdf [accessed Oct. 2, 2002].

MEDSTAT. 1998. *A Guide for States to Assist in the Collection and Analysis of Medicaid Managed Care Data (CMS Contract #500-92-0035).* Baltimore: CMS.

Mencke, N. M., L. G. Alley, and J. Etchason. 2000. Application of HEDIS measures within a Veterans Affairs medical center. *Am J Manag Care* 6 (6):661-8.

Milbank Memorial Fund. 2001. "Value Purchasers in Health Care: Seven Case Studies; The Military Health System: Implementing a Vision for Value." Online. Available at http://www.milbank.org/2001ValuePurchasers/011001valuepurchasers.html#military [accessed May 14, 2002].

Nerenz, D. R., and N. Neil. 2001. "Performance Measures for Health Care Systems, Commissioned Paper for the Center for Health Management Research." Online. Available at http://depts.washington.edu/chmr/docs/commissioned_papers/performance measures_nerenz_2001.doc [accessed June 14, 2002].

Paul, B. (CMS). 8 August 2002. BIPA 2000. Personal communication to Jill Eden.

Quality Interagency Coordination. 2002. "Quality Interagency Coordination (QuIC) Task Force." Online. Available at http://www.quic.gov/index.htm [accessed July 11, 2002].

Rhew, D. C., M. B. Goetz, and P. G. Shekelle. 2001. Evaluating quality indicators for patients with community-acquired pneumonia. *Jt Comm J Qual Improv* 27 (11):575-90.

Roper, W. L., and C. M. Cutler. 1998. Health plan accountability and reporting: issues and challenges. *Health Aff (Millwood)* 17 (2):152-5.

Rubin, H. R., P. Pronovost, and G. B. Diette. 2001. The advantages and disadvantages of process-based measures of health care quality. *Int J Qual Health Care* 13 (6):469-74.

Schneider, E. C., V. Riehl, S. Courte-Wienecke, D. M. Eddy, and C. Sennett. 1999. Enhancing performance measurement: NCQA's road map for a health information framework. National Committee for Quality Assurance. *JAMA* 282 (12):1184-90.

Shaughnessy, P. W., D. F. Hittle, K. S. Crisler, M. C. Powell, A. A. Richard, A. M. Kramer, R. E. Schlenker, J. F. Steiner, N. S. Donelan-McCall, J. M. Beaudry, K. L. Mulvey-Lawlor, and K. Engle. 2002. Improving patient outcomes of home health care: findings from two demonstration trials of outcome-based quality improvement. *J Am Geriatr Soc* 50 (8):1354-64.

Shukri, K., J. Henderson, and W. Daley. 2002. The comparative assessment and improvement of quality of surgical care in the Department of Veteran's Affairs. *Arch Surg* 137:20-27.

Sofaer, S. 2002. Why ask patients? Presentation at the annual meeting of the Academy for Health Services Research and Health Policy, Washington DC.

Stuber, J., G. Dallek, and B. Biles. 2001. *Program on Medicare's Future: National and local factors driving health plan withdrawals from Medicare+Choice.* New York: The Commonwealth Fund.

Texas Medical Foundation. 2002. "Diabetes quality improvement project." Online. Available at www.dqip.org [accessed July 10, 2002].

TRICARE. 1999a. "Health Care Survey of DOD Beneficiaries: Overview." Online. Available at http://www.tricare.osd.mil/survey/hcsurvey/overview.html [accessed May 13, 2002a].

———. 1999b. "MHS Optimization Plan February 1999 Interim Report." Online. Available at http://www.tricare.osd.mil/mhsophsc/mhs_supportcenter/Library/MHS_Optimization_Plan.pdf [accessed May 14, 2002b].

Verdier, J., and R. Dodge. 2002. *Other Data Sources and Uses, Working Paper in the Informed Purchasing Series.* Lawrenceville NJ: Center for Health Care Strategies.

5

Building Stronger
Information Capabilities

Summary of Chapter Recommendations

As discussed in Chapter 4, the Committee recommends that by 2005, all health care providers participating in government health care programs be capable of electronically gathering and reporting the subset of patient-level data needed to calculate the core sets of performance measures. Full implementation of this recommendation will depend in part on the development of a more sophisticated clinical information technology infrastructure throughout the health care system.

RECOMMENDATION 5: The federal government should take steps immediately to encourage and facilitate the development of the information technology infrastructure that is critical to health care quality and safety enhancement, as well as to many of the nation's other priorities, such as bioterrorism surveillance, public health, and research. Specifically:

a. Congress should consider potential options to facilitate rapid development of a national health information infrastructure, including tax credits, subsidized loans, and grants.
b. Government health care programs that deliver services through the private sector—Medicare, Medicaid, the State Children's Health Insurance Program (SCHIP), and a portion of Department of Defense (DOD) TRICARE—should adopt both market-based and regulatory options to encourage investment in information technology. Such options might include enhanced or more rapid payments to providers capable of submitting computerized clinical data, a requirement for certain information technology capabilities as a condition of participation, and direct grants.

c. **The Veterans Health Administration (VHA), DOD TRICARE, and the Indian Health Service (IHS) should continue implementing clinical and administrative information systems that enable the retrieval of clinical information across their programs and can communicate directly with each other. Whenever possible, the software and intellectual property developed by these three government programs should rely on Web-based language and architecture and be made available in the public domain.**

Although this report focuses on the federal government's role, the committee believes private-sector purchasers should also contribute to building the country's health information infrastructure by providing financial and other incentives.

Comparative quality data should be available in the public domain for use by many stakeholders. There are numerous potential uses of such data. Public- and private-sector oversight organizations might rely on performance measurement data to develop benchmarks for the clinical practice patterns of providers and goals for stimulating improvements in clinical care. The data would also be useful to states and communities as a way of monitoring the progress of community-based efforts in meeting public health goals (e.g., reducing obesity and use of tobacco). Professional groups, including board certification entities and others involved in continuing education, would be likely to use the data to provide ongoing feedback to providers and identify best practices. Group purchasers and consumers might use the quality data to assist in the selection of providers and health plans.

RECOMMENDATION 6: Starting in FY 2008, each government health care program should make comparative quality reports and data available in the public domain. The programs should provide for access to these reports and data in ways that meet the needs of various users, provided that patient privacy is protected.

Pooling of performance data across all six major government programs would enable more accurate performance assessment for those receiving services through multiple programs. It would also permit benchmarking of performance levels across programs.

RECOMMENDATION 7: The government health care programs, working with the Agency for Healthcare Research and Quality (AHRQ), should establish a mechanism for pooling performance measurement data across programs in a data repository. Contributions of data from private-sector insurance programs should be encouraged provided such data meet certain standards for validity and reliability. Consumers, health care professionals, planners, purchasers, regulators, public health officials, researchers, and others should be afforded access to the repository, provided that patient privacy is protected.

The committee is recommending a strategy for quality enhancement that relies on measurement and reporting of standardized performance measures across the government health care programs. Valid clinical performance measurement depends on the availability of clinical data (McGlynn and Brook, 2001).

Access to data remains problematic in a health care system that still depends largely on claims data, abstraction of data from paper records, and surveys to determine whether patients are receiving identified elements of care. The dependence on abstraction generally limits performance measurement to evaluation of entities with sufficient administrative infrastructure to develop the necessary data, such as hospitals, health plans, and large group practices, thereby excluding many small ambulatory care settings where a large proportion of care is delivered. Record abstraction is a labor-intensive process that usually occurs retrospectively rather than as an integral part of the clinical process, imposing a burden that prohibits more than intermittent review. While less costly than record abstraction, reliance on claims data may not provide the level of clinical detail required to track processes of care accurately (McIntyre et al., 2001; Schneider and Lieberman, 2001). For example, current claims data in many cases do not indicate whether complications in the course of hospitalization arose from preexisting comorbidities or adverse consequences of care. Moreover, claims data are available only for insured populations and are limited to billable services, thus constraining the aspects of care that can be evaluated.

Today's data sources simply cannot support the strategy for quality enhancement proposed in this report. Indeed, there is broad consensus that the nation must develop a functional health care information technology infrastructure (Becher and Chassin, 2001; Eddy, 1998; Institute of Medicine, 2001; McGlynn and Brook, 2001; National Committee on Vital and Health Statistics, 2001; Schneider et al., 1999). Growing evidence supports the conclusion that automated clinical information and decision-support systems are critical to addressing the nation's health care quality gap (Institute of Medicine, 2001). Computerized order entry and electronic medical records have been found to result in measurably improved care and better outcomes for patients (Bates et al., 1999; Birkmeyer et al., 2002; Webster, 2001). These results are particularly notable when electronic ordering triggers clinical decision-support information, for example, on antibiotic use (Christakis et al., 2001; Demakis et al., 2000; Rollman et al., 2001; Safran, 2001). Similar evidence suggests that these systems have the potential to reduce costs as well (Birkmeyer et al., 2002; Webster, 2001). In one study in which electronic order entry was accompanied by decision-support tools such as allergy and drug-interaction warnings, serious medication errors were demonstrated to decline by 86 percent (Bates et al.,

1999). Anecdotal reporting on the experience of individual hospitals confirms significant error reduction and savings in labor costs (Landro, 2002; Webster, 2001). Other experiments in the use of technology to improve outcomes and increase efficiency are ongoing. For example, an element of some of the Medicare Coordinated Care Demonstration Projects discussed in Chapter 3 is to evaluate the impact of electronic remote monitoring of patients to manage treatment (Department of Health and Human Services, 2001; Georgetown University Medical Center, 2002). While it may be too early to determine whether the observed cost savings completely offset or exceed the costs of setting up such systems, evidence on the reduction in harm to patients from computerized order entry is unambiguous and significant (Birkmeyer et al., 2002).

Standardized performance measure datasets containing patient-level information could be mined to learn many things and to support various strategies for quality improvement. Providers could use comparative quality data to benchmark their performance and share information on best practices. Groups such as the American Board of Medical Specialties and many of its member boards, which are already expanding practice oversight activities as an integral component of their recertification processes, may use the data as an input to decision-making (American Board of Medical Specialties, 2000). Government programs would be able to identify the levels of care received by different populations served by a program, such as rural and urban populations or those residing in different regions; they could then target strategies to address those disparities. Such datasets could also support the development of targeted regulatory strategies, such as reduced regulatory burden for providers that achieve quality goals or intensified participation in quality improvement initiatives for providers whose performance was determined to be substandard.

Uniform automated datasets also offer the opportunity for government programs to develop multiple formats for the presentation of performance data tailored to the needs of specific audiences, including providers, consumers, and community health care leaders (Hibbard et al., 2002). Reporting efforts for consumers should recognize the diversity of cultural, racial, and ethnic groups being served, including differences in languages and levels of health literacy. Quality reports for providers should be tailored to assist clinicians in identifying opportunities for improvement in their own practices. Efforts should also be made to provide physicians with information that can better inform their referrals of patients to specialists and hospitals.

As discussed in Chapter 4, providers and plans are faced with a multiplicity of measures from a variety of sources with which they have varying relationships, adding to the burden of a cumbersome collection process. In addition, current performance measurement fails to capture how providers interact across settings and organizations in providing care to individuals (Paone, 2001). This weakness reflects underlying limitations in the ability of providers to communicate with each other regarding patient care or to have real-time access to information on concurrent treatment of individual patients by multiple providers. Tracking clinical performance requires an integrated health information framework (Schneider et al., 1999). That framework depends in turn on the development of computerized clinical data (Gawande and Bates, 2000; McGlynn and Brook, 2001; McIntyre et al., 2001; Schneider et al., 1999).

The remainder of this chapter reviews the current status of information technology development in the government health care programs, examines strategies for motivating the development of enhanced capabilities, and addresses the key issue of access to the resulting information.

THE STATUS OF INFORMATION TECHNOLOGY DEVELOPMENT

The integration of information technology into health care beyond administrative and billing transactions is a complex task. The design of an information technology system and the way in which its components are connected to and operate with each other is referred to as the system *architecture*. An adequate information technology infrastructure requires an architecture that links and distributes robust clinical information throughout the network while also meeting the information and technology needs of specific users. In addition, health care organizations must meet the growing interest among patients in online access to their health information and the technology applications that can assist them with distance care (Rundle, 2002). Moreover, such applications must be consistent with the privacy protections in the Health Insurance Portability and Accountability Act (HIPAA; Public Law 104-191).

Significant technical and financial barriers have impeded electronic infrastructure development in the private health care sector. Creation of an IT infrastructure requires capital investment and ongoing resources for system maintenance. Initial implementation of systems may also entail disruptions in practice, and temporary loss of practice revenues. In the current environment, incentives to providers to make the necessary investments are lacking, and this lack of financial incentives is compounded by technical barriers that cause many providers to question the value of the investment.

The development of robust infrastructures for information technology in the health care arena has been hampered by a lack of national standards for the coding and classification of clinical and other health care data and the transmission and sharing of such data (National Committee on Vital and Health Statistics, 2001). Numerous efforts are underway to address this issue including: 1) the Consolidated Health Informatics Initiative, created under the auspices of the White House Office of Management and Budget in 2001 to facilitate the development of standards that would ensure compatible information technology systems across the government health programs (Office of Management and Budget, 2002); 2) the Markle Foundation's Connecting for Health Initiative (2002); and 3) an IOM project on Patient Safety Data Standards. It is important that these initiatives move forward expeditiously to address the critical need for national data standards.

It should be noted that the establishment of national standardized performance measures by the federal government in collaboration with the private sector, as recommended in this report, will remove one major barrier to the development of clinical data standards. The lack of clarity and consistency in performance reporting requirements across public and private payers and other stakeholders currently complicates efforts to reach a broad-based consensus around the content and representation of clinical data elements. The forthcoming IOM report on patient safety data standards will be addressing this issue in greater detail.

There are differences in information technology infrastructures across the six major government programs. In general, the four government programs that pay for health care delivered through the private sector—Medicare, Medicaid, SCHIP, and a portion of the DOD TRICARE program—have limited ability to obtain computerized clinical data from providers, reflecting the low level of automation in this sector. By contrast, the government health care programs characterized by government ownership and operation of the direct care system—the programs of VHA and IHS, and the remainder of DOD TRICARE—have implemented more computerized clinical data systems and decision-support applications.

Government Programs That Deliver Care Through the Private Sector

As noted, Medicare, Medicaid, SCHIP, and a portion of TRICARE provide care to beneficiaries through the private sector. Accordingly, their clinical data capacity largely mirrors the limited applications of information technology in most private-sector health care delivery settings. These government programs primarily collect claims and encounter data from which some clinical data can be mined.

For Medicaid and Medicare managed care, the Health Plan Employer Data and Information Set (HEDIS) and other data can be obtained at the health plan level for specified conditions and quality improvement projects, and data can be gathered from medical chart abstraction and audits of Quality Improvement Organizations (QIOs) in the fee-for-service (FFS) sector (MacTaggart, 2002). In addition, Medicaid maintains the Medicaid Management Information System, a hardware and software system that enables the states to collect claims and encounter data and submit them to the federal government in the form of the Medicaid Statistical Information Set (MSIS). These systems are designed to track utilization rather than provide clinical data for performance measurement (Friedman, 2002). MSIS provides patient-level data, but it does not include data on providers. Patient-level data available at the state level are not shared with CMS (Buchanan, 2002). CMS receives summary, aggregate reports from states. The capacity to gather computerized clinical data from the majority of clinicians in sufficient detail to enable performance measurement remains largely undeveloped.

Government Programs That Provide Direct Care

The largest programs that provide direct care—that of the VHA and that portion of TRICARE provided by DOD through its own facilities and infrastructure (the Military Health System)[1] —have developed systems for recording and extracting clinical data that stem from their adoption of the computer-based patient record. IHS has developed substantial automated clinical data capacity that complements medical chart abstraction entered electronically, instead of relying on a computer-based patient record.

Veterans Health Administration

VHA has one of the largest integrated health information systems in the United States. Its operating objective is to input data once that can be utilized throughout the network by different types of users on an authorized basis. This system enables electronic documentation of health data, real-time access to important clinical information at the point of care (e.g., radiological images, laboratory test results, clinical observations, and pharmacy orders), and linkages to facilitate administrative and financial processing. Other applications such as those for reporting adverse medical events represent spearheading efforts to use health information systems to improve patient safety. A technical description of the VHA system is provided in Appendix C.

At the heart of the VHA health information system is the Computerized Patient Record System (CPRS) which serves as a unifying platform

---

[1]For the purposes of this chapter, the Military Health System refers to those services and facilities directly owned and operated by the government as opposed to care that is purchased from the private sector.

for the integration of all patient-oriented applications (e.g., administrative, clinical) across the network. The current CPRS is a Windows-type desktop program that displays all relevant patient data needed to support clinical decision making. It enables clinicians to enter, review, and continuously update all information (including pharmacy, laboratory, and radiology) related to any patient. The CPRS can also be accessed from the operating room and enables automatic generation of the postoperative report. To address privacy concerns, access to CPRS is limited to those authorized to perform various actions on specific clinical documents. The system depends on a legacy server with limited portability for other users. However, VHA is in the process of upgrading to a system that uses Web-based language. VHA's information technology upgrade is expected to be completed by 2005 (Christopherson, 2002). The projected costs associated with the upgrade are approximately $100 million in 2002 and $150 million in 2003 (Christopherson, 2002).

In addition to provider-oriented applications of medical records for gathering clinical data, VHA has established the *My Healthy Vet* program, which provides veterans an online connection to their medical records. Participating veterans can obtain electronic copies of key portions of their electronic health records, add medical information in a "self-entered" section, and link to a health education library.

The Military Health System

The MHS provides information technology support to over 540 military facilities worldwide. A brief technical description of the MHS information systems and their applications is provided in Appendix C.

Like VHA, the MHS currently maintains a computerized patient record (CPR) for laboratory, radiology, and pharmacy information. By the end of 2002, it will launch a pilot of a fully electronic CPR that will establish an individual's medical record from beginning to end of military service. The record will be linked to a Clinical Data Repository (CDR) that currently serves as a "clinical warehouse" for electronic laboratory, radiology, and pharmacy data, and for applications associated with the CPR (e.g., wellness alerts, provider prompts). Data in the CDR will support clinical research, wellness alerts, symptom surveillance, and population health improvement efforts.

The Theater Medical Information Program (TMIP) provides data for the clinical care of battlefield casualties and the management of military medical assets. TMIP functions on an independent temporary database system that is linked to a clinical data repository—the Composite Health Care System. During deployment, the relevant medical information in a patient's electronic record (held in the CDR) is accessed through TMIP.

All clinical documentation related to local treatment during deployment is held in the temporary database. Upon the return of the force personnel, the new medical information is downloaded into the CDR and the patient's CPR.

Scheduled for roll-out to all facilities in late 2002, the military's e-health communications system, TRICARE Online, will provide information to patients on health conditions and interactive health tools, disease management and treatment compliance recommendations, TRICARE medical facilities and providers, and appointment scheduling. Patients will be able to create their own personal health care home page to store medical information and resources in a secure environment.

The various elements of the VHA and MHS systems are designed to integrate clinical care activities with quality enhancement and measurement. Accordingly, clinicians are not required to create or participate in separate processes to gather data, file reports, and address quality concerns. Rather, relevant information can be retrieved automatically for a variety of different purposes. The result is a system that is less burdensome and supports clinical care across multiple settings.

Indian Health Service

IHS has developed an automated system of patient-level clinical data for its outpatient facilities that is used to support care delivery and to provide the capacity to conduct performance measurement. Radiology images and results, laboratory tests, and prescription orders are entered electronically in a patient-specific field. Paper medical charts are routinely abstracted in the medical records department of the facility and added to the electronic records as the Patient Care Component (PCC), a process that necessarily entails redundant labor and delay in the electronic inclusion of clinical care data. The abstracted PCC data include date and time of visit, provider identification, vital statistics, diagnosis, treatment modalities, patient education efforts, and surgical and injury history. The electronic information system employs multiple clinical applications of the PCC, such as triggers to decision-support tools, summaries of the 10 most recent encounters, and graphed laboratory values. The system can produce data on performance measures and respond to aggregate queries. While the electronic system is integrated at the site of care, it is not fully integrated across the different sites within the IHS system. A subset of the PCC data is transmitted to the central data warehouse maintained by IHS—the National Patient Information Reporting System (Kihega, 2002).

Joint Information Technology Initiatives

In May 2002, as the result of a White House initiative in 1997–98 to better track the course of apparent service-connected disease processes following the Gulf War, VHA and DOD began operating the Federal Health Information Exchange (FHIE). FHIE allows each program to send designated clinical information, such as pharmacy and laboratory data to a common database and retrieve data submitted by the other program as needed (Christopherson, 2002). The second phase of the joint operation is expected to be completed in 2006, after DOD finishes instituting its electronic medical record system. This phase will result in implementation of electronic information systems that are compatible between VHA and DOD and that will be able to communicate directly with each other without having to go through a common database. In addition, it is anticipated that IHS and VHA will coordinate on clinical software development for future applications. Supporting the above efforts will be the previously mentioned Consolidated Health Informatics initiative to develop common clinical data standards under the leadership of the Centers for Medicare and Medicaid Services (CMS) (Christopherson, 2002). Such common standards would enhance the usefulness and dissemination of the VHA/DOD technology to other programs and the private sector.

MOTIVATING CHANGE

The committee is recommending that each of the government health care programs implement a core set of standardized performance measures by 2005, and that the number of measures be steadily increased over the next 5 to 8 years (see Chapter 4). Provider reporting of data necessary to enable performance measurement is required by 2007. Although it may be possible in the short run for government programs that deliver care through the private sector to rely on medical record abstraction to meet this requirement, greater computerization of clinical information will be required over the long run to sustain performance measurement, apply it to a broader range of conditions, and decrease the associated administrative burden on providers. It is anticipated that each of the government programs will pursue different strategies for stimulating the development of enhanced information technology capabilities. The challenges clearly will be much greater for those programs that deliver care through the private sector. However, programs that provide direct care will also need to make some changes. For all programs, the assurance of substantial and effective privacy protections for patient-level data is essential to the support needed by both providers and patients to make the collection of data for performance measurement operational.

Fostering Information Technology Development
in the Private Health Care Sector

For providers that currently rely on computers simply for billing and appointment scheduling, building a clinical data capacity will require both capital and training investments. It is the committee's conclusion that motivating providers associated with government programs to undertake the changes necessary for quality enhancement will require incentives and assistance. A range of actions—from payment and contracting incentives to tax credits and direct grants to regulation—are available to generate change. The committee encourages each government health care program to evaluate these options, sponsor private/public collaboration on the best approaches to development, and select those most appropriate to its objectives.

Financial and Administrative Incentives

To offset the costs of the capital investment and training required to achieve greater levels of automation, higher payments could be offered to providers that can harvest and submit clinical data electronically according to standardized core sets of clinical performance measures. Alternatively, those that submit performance data electronically could receive more rapid electronic payment. In Medicaid and SCHIP, direct financial incentives could be instituted through a substantially enhanced match to states to make payments to providers that meet certain automation standards. Contractors that meet specified information technology capacity could also be eligible for bonuses or other financial rewards (Kaye and Bailit, 1999). In addition, the government health programs could identify regulatory or administrative requirements that could be waived for providers with specified electronic capabilities.

While the above approaches can be expected to entice some providers to meet new electronic standards, they still leave providers substantial discretion to maintain the status quo. Other means of fostering change may therefore be necessary.

Contracting and Regulation

To accelerate the adoption of clinical information systems, program contracts with providers could include standardized information technology specifications as a contract condition. Similar provisions included in Medicaid contracts with managed care organizations require specified administrative data capacity, quality improvement activities, and grievance and appeal procedures (Rosenbaum et al., 1998).

Consistent with the recommendations in Chapter 4, providers could be required as a condition of participation (COP) to make available in automated form, by specified dates, the clinical data needed for performance measurement, with standardized data elements, definitions, and terminology. The advantage of making specified levels of information technology capability a contract term or COP is that it would eliminate provider discretion to continue existing practices, apply to all providers equally, and ensure that all populations would benefit equally from quality enhancement activities. The disadvantage is that without increased payments, such a requirement could exact a disproportionate outlay from safety net providers with strained resources, resulting in unintended negative effects on access to care.

Alternatively, maintenance of automated data could be a condition of payment. As a practical matter, this approach would motivate providers to automate clinical data as quickly as a COP. However, it raises similar concerns about the effects on safety net providers and access to care. Accordingly, any regulatory contracting strategy to improve provider information technology capabilities should be accompanied by appropriate financial support for such providers.

Grants and Tax Credits

The committee envisions a health information infrastructure that enables transfer of the information necessary to measure care across settings, time, and programs to reflect the needs and care experiences of patients, rather than the silo functions of individual providers. Such an infrastructure implies a transformation in the care delivery process that requires national commitment. The Hill-Burton Act (Public Law 79-725) established a grant and loan program that subsidizes construction costs to increase hospital capacity, contributing over $6 billion to that effort in the private sector (Health Resources and Services Administration, 2000). A similar substantial grant program should be considered to assure the proliferation of an information technology infrastructure that can ultimately support clinical care and enable performance measurement as a seamless process. Such a program could be initiated with targeted demonstration projects testing the amount, structure, and effectiveness of the grants, as well as their applicability to different types of providers.

Each program will need to conduct its own analysis of the most effective strategies for motivating change among its participating providers while collaborating with the other programs to ensure complementary approaches. It is the committee's expectation that a combination of approaches, such as higher payments to safety net or other providers and direct grants combined with information technology–related conditions of participation, payment, and contracting, would achieve the highest level of information technology improvement in the shortest amount of time with the least effect on access. While the committee recognizes that the initial investment required is large, the benefits of preventing errors, improving care and health status, and reducing duplication of services that can accrue from real-time access to current clinical information will offset much of the cost and provide a substantial public good. Beyond quality improvement, a robust health information infrastructure is essential to other national priorities, such as the medical tracking and follow-up critical to identifying and combating bioterrorism. Support for development of an adequate clinical information technology infrastructure should be commensurate with its importance to domestic security.

Information Technology Development in Direct Care Programs

While the largest government providers, VHA and the MHS, have a significant record of accomplishment and ongoing commitment to innovation in their systems, implementation of the committee's recommendations will require that they move rapidly to complete the standardization and compatibility efforts now in process, and to ensure that such standardization is amenable to Web-based applications and dissemination to the private sector. VHA is currently reconfiguring its information technology system to make data definitions conform to Web-based language. This reconfiguration should support implementation of the standardized core datasets needed for performance measurement. The MHS needs to complete the expansion of its system to all regions and develop strategies for including clinical data from care delivered through its external purchased network in its health information system.

In all the programs in which the government is the direct provider of care, investments should be made in information technology infrastructure appropriate to the needs of the programs. It was the direct government investments in information technology infrastructure that led to the VHA systems. This infrastructure is now regarded by the clinicians using it as indispensable to direct care, even though it requires new investment for essential updating. Proportionate investments should be made to ensure the development of compatible information technology systems in public health and community clinics and in IHS.

The ongoing collaborative efforts of VHA, the MHS, IHS, and CMS to develop uniform systems are supported by the programs' discretionary funds and have received no specific financial support from Congress (Christopherson, 2002). As a result of its size, scope, and range of applications, however, information technology collaboration among the federal programs provides the foundation for development of an electronic infrastructure with the strongest potential for dissemination. Accordingly, it is the committee's conclusion that additional funding will likely be needed to ensure the full implementation of uniform, compatible federal health information technology that lends itself easily to private-sector applications in the spirit of technology transfer from the government.

As the history of the Internet illustrates, the proliferation of electronic capacity among large numbers of providers creates its own momentum, driving the expansion of usage among others not previously engaged (Gladwell, 2000). The surmountable financial, organizational, and inertia challenges to building an information technology infrastructure in the health care sector are apparent. Given the demonstrated need for effective quality enhancement activities, however. it is equally clear that the status quo is not acceptable.

ACCESS TO INFORMATION

It is the committee's conclusion that improving public access to information on health care quality will increase the impetus for addressing safety and quality concerns and is an important component of a comprehensive strategy to achieve significant improvement in the coming decade. Improving consumers' awareness of the variability in the quality of health care is a necessary prerequisite to engaging them in making choices based on quality. Public access to such information has the potential to drive consumers to select better care, while also giving providers incentives to improve care (Marshall et al., 2000), furnishing accrediting boards and certifying entities with additional information and tools to motivate improved clinical care, and facilitating community and public health planning.

Overview of Reporting Efforts

To date, public reporting efforts have focused primarily on health plans, and to a lesser degree, hospitals or particular surgical interventions (Schauffler and Mordavsky, 2001). Very limited comparative information has been released for medical groups or physicians.

Most health plan report cards include process of care measures (HEDIS), patient perceptions of care (CAHPS), and accreditation status (McGlynn and Adams, 2001; National Committee for Quality Assurance, 2002). Analyses of impact have consistently found that such report cards have little impact on consumer decision-making (Schauffler and Mordavsky, 2001). Many factors appear to contribute to the lack of impact (Hibbard et al., 2001; Hibbard, 1998; McGlynn and Adams, 2001; Schauffler and Mordavsky, 2001), including:

1. The decision of most relevance to consumers is the selection of a provider not a health plan, probably in part, because many consumers have very limited choice of health plans.

2. The performance measures do not reflect issues of importance to consumers, but rather, what it is easy to measure given existing administrative data sets.

3. The information presented is too complex for most consumers to understand.

4. There is too much information for most consumers to process and use.

5. The report cards are not produced by a trusted source.

6. Consumers were not aware of the existence of the report cards.

Report cards focusing on hospitals or procedures are even less in number and there is very limited evidence regarding impact. For example, there is evidence that report cards, in combination with other interventions, have stimulated specific clinical changes to improve care among the poorest-performing providers in cardiac surgery in New York (Chassin, 2002; Hannan et al., 1994, 1997).

Comparative quality reporting is a rapidly developing trend in both the public and private health care sectors, to a great extent in response to growing demand for information on the quality of care (California HealthCare Foundation, 2002). In addition to CMS' publication of comparative information on nursing homes, dialysis centers, and health plans, business groups and health plans have begun making public comparative surveys of consumer satisfaction with provider groups. For example, the Pacific Business Group on Health, Pacificare, HealthNet, and Blue Cross of California each put out separate proprietary report cards on their participating provider groups, many of whom overlap between plans. The Health Resources and Services Administration (HRSA) sponsors a Website that compares kidney transplant outcomes by provider across the nation (Scientific Registry of Transplant Recipients, 2001). A growing number of states, including New York, Pennsylvania, and California, publish annually the comparative outcomes by provider of cardiac bypass surgery. In addition to cardiac bypass surgery reports, the Pennsylvania Health Care Cost Containment Council puts out comparative reports on hospital and health plan performance and maintains several interactive databases that users can access to generate their own quality reports (Pennsylvania Health Care Cost Containment Council, 2002). There are numerous hospital surveys including the Leapfrog Hospital Survey, the California Hospital Outcomes Program, and the Patients' Evaluation of Performance in California. Many of these surveys capture experiences that represent important patient-centered dimensions of quality that may not be reflected in more clinical performance measures such as respect for patient preferences, coordination of care, pain relief, and emotional support (California HealthCare Foundation, 2002).

While the need for research to improve the efficacy, accuracy, and salience of comparative reports is discussed in some detail in Chapter 6, the proliferation of comparative reporting provides a distinct opportunity for leadership from the government health programs. Specifically, the standardization of definitions, sampling techniques and other methodologies, and statistical analysis could improve significantly the consistency of survey findings and assure the apples-to-apples comparisons that are currently lacking in many of these efforts (McGlynn et al., 1999; Simon and Monroe, 2001). Such standardization also would reduce the burden on provider groups who must respond to multiple surveys and audits and deal with inconsistent ratings provided by diverse purchasers/plans (Simon and Monroe, 2001). The committee believes that collaboration between those private entities with experience with provider-level report cards and the government health programs would facilitate the necessary standardization to achieve reliability, burden reduction, and greater dissemination of information on quality of care.

In summary, public reporting initiatives are in an early stage of development. To date, the quality measures and reports that have been provided to consumers appear not to have captured their interest. Yet the evidence is sparse and mixed, thus it must be interpreted cautiously. Reporting efforts with sufficient clinical detail for providers are even fewer in number, but here there are some promising results. Accreditation and certification entities are actively engaged in the collection, and in some cases reporting, of comparative performance data, and the National Committee for Quality Assurance (NCQA), in particular, has been a leader in this area. Indeed, performance measurement has become an integral part of most leading private sector oversight processes. It seems likely that these groups would make use of richer comparative data as it becomes available, especially if they are involved as partners in the developmental efforts.

Program Transparency

The IOM Committee has concluded, like an earlier IOM committee (Institute of Medicine, 2001: Chapter 3), that steps should be taken to make performance measurement data available to various stakeholders in ways that will be most useful. It is unclear the extent to which various stakeholders will use these data, because most reporting efforts to date have been poorly designed and executed and hampered by the absence of detailed clinical data to derive measures likely to be meaningful to various users. Consequently, future reporting efforts should be carefully designed, pilot tested and evaluated and subject to continuous refinement.

The steady demand for comparative performance data by accrediting entities, group purchasers, health plans, state governments, and others is indicative of a keen interest in quality information. If the federal government does not share performance measurement data and information with private sector stakeholders, it is very likely that these groups will continue to impose their own reporting requirements on providers, thus contributing to administrative burden.

Comparative data could be made available through prepared reports that synthesize data according to subjects or themes, authorized queries of the database, or analysis of data displayed on Websites. The data available should enable users to determine the comparative performance of providers or groups of providers in a program, as well as the program's performance in improving quality of care. For program operation purposes, comparative data should enable the establishment of valid baselines within programs and the assessment of improvement or deterioration in performance. In addition, comparative data analysis will enable programs to assess geographic and population-specific disparities in care, as well as program-wide patterns of deficiency. For example, such analysis could reveal racial disparities within programs or disparities in care between Medicare and Medicaid.

Accordingly, program-level data should be susceptible to analysis for a range of purposes by a variety of users. The programs should be able to receive, store, and organize the data into domains appropriate for different types of users, such as consumers, purchasers, providers, regulators and their contractors, the public health community, researchers, and policy makers. The program database should be structured to provide different levels of access to data depending on the decision needs of the user.

Once comparative clinical measures are available, they can be used as tools in the government's multiple roles in its health programs—purchaser, regulator, and provider. To enhance the effectiveness of regulation in bringing specific benefits to the public, the performance data can aid regulators in identifying substandard performance and developing cross-program strategies for improving care. To improve market performance in achieving quality goals, comparative data can inform purchasers (including government purchasers) in the selection and payment of contractors based on clinical performance.

As a market tool for consumers, access to information on the comparative quality performance of different providers for the core sets of measures, according to consistent standards and methodologies, is essential. Comparative data appropriately presented have the potential to assist consumers in provider and plan selection, thereby creating market incentives for providers to improve care as well as channeling patients to higher quality providers as reflected by the measures. Similarly, access by providers (including government operated delivery systems) to comparative information on quality may enable them to better assess their own clinical environment and identify accepted processes for improving care.

The provision of comparative performance data to patients may also provide the opportunity to educate patients about the critical elements of their care. While the effect of performance measures on patients' medical self-management has not been evaluated, familiarity with the core measures could potentially enable consumers to better understand the critical elements of their care and become more active participants in their own health care management (Greenfield et al., 1985). For example, familiarity with diabetes process measures could stimulate diabetic patients to request eye exams or track their level of blood sugar control. Finally, comparative performance data could augment existing public health mechanisms for tracking the incidence and prevalence of certain types of diseases and interventions.

Use of a Pooled Data Repository Across Programs

The government programs should explore mechanisms for pooling the performance data needed to evaluate and compare quality across populations and programs. Pooled data could support quality enhancement at both the micro and macro levels; pooled Diabetes Quality Improvement (DQIP) data, for example, can help identify geographic, provider-level, and program-specific variations in the quality of diabetes care.

Private entities could also participate in the data repository, as long as they satisfy safeguards to assure data validity and reliability. The ability afforded by such a pool to enable broader, more population-based comparisons gives private plans an incentive to participate both to improve provider selection and evaluate their own performance.

The Agency for Healthcare Research and Quality (AHRQ) is well positioned to work with participating programs in developing and managing a pooled data repository. In designing the repository, AHRQ should get consumer and other stakeholder input. AHRQ's research orientation provides the technical and analytical expertise needed to assess the validity of data to develop reporting and data access strategies to meet the needs of various users. In establishing the repository, AHRQ will need to assure compliance with HIPAA requirements for patient privacy. It is anticipated that any patient-level data would be stripped of identifiers.

REFERENCES

American Board of Medical Specialties. 2000. "ABMS Home Page." Online. Available at http://www.abms.org/ [accessed Sept. 30, 2002].

Bates, D. W., J. M. Teich, J. Lee, D. Seger, G. J. Kuperman, N. Ma'Luf, D. Boyle, and L. Leape. 1999. The impact of computerized physician order entry on medication error prevention. *J Am Med Inform Assoc* 6 (4):313-21.

Becher, E. C., and M. R. Chassin. 2001. Improving quality, minimizing error: making it happen. *Health Aff (Millwood)* 20 (3):68-81.

Birkmeyer, C. M., J. Lee, D. W. Bates, and J. D. Birkmeyer. 2002. Will electronic order entry reduce health care costs? *Eff Clin Pract* 5:67-74.

Buchanan, R. (CMS). 3 May 2002. Personal communication to Jill Eden.

California HealthCare Foundation. 2002. "Quality Nears Tipping Point in California: Accountability Efforts Multiply." Online. Available at http://www.chcf.org/topics/view.cfm?itemID=19764 [accessed Sept. 6, 2002].

Chassin, M. 2002. Achieving and sustaining improved quality: lessons from New York state and cardiac surgery. *Health Aff (Millwood)* 21 (4):40-51.

Christakis, D. A., F. J. Zimmerman, J. A. Wright, M. M. Garrison, F. P. Rivara, and R. L. Davis. 2001. A randomized controlled trial of point-of-care evidence to improve the antibiotic prescribing practices for otitis media in children. *Pediatrics* 107 (2):E15.

Christopherson, G. (VHA). 6 June 2002. Personal communication to Barbara Smith.

Demakis, J. G., C. Beauchamp, W. L. Cull, R. Denwood, S. A. Eisen, R. Lofgren, K. Nichol, J. Woolliscroft, and W. G. Henderson. 2000. Improving residents' compliance with standards of ambulatory care: results from the VA Cooperative Study on Computerized Reminders. *JAMA* 284 (11):1411-16.

Department of Health and Human Services. 2001. *Medicare Fact Sheet: Providing Coordinated Care to Improve Quality of Care for Chronically Ill Medicare Beneficiaries.* Washington DC: U.S. Department of Health and Human Services.

Eddy, D. M. 1998. Performance measurement: problems and solutions. *Health Aff (Millwood)* 17 (4):7-25 .

Friedman, R. (CMS). 14 May 2002. Personal communication to Barbara Smith.

Gawande, A. A., and D. W. Bates. 2000. The use of information technology in improving medical performance. Part I. Information systems for medical transactions. *MedGenMed* Feb. 7:E14.

Georgetown University Medical Center. 2002. "The Imaging Science and Information Systems (ISIS) Center." Online. Available at http://www.imac.georgetown.edu/aboutisis/research.htm [accessed Sept. 4, 2002].

Gladwell, M. 2000. *The Tipping Point: How Little Things Can Make a Big Difference.* Boston: Little, Brown, and Co.

Greenfield, S., S. Kaplan, and J. E. J. Ware. 1985. Expanding patient involvement in care. Effects on patient outcomes. *Ann Intern Med* 102 (4):520-8.

Hannan, E., H. Kilburn, M. Racz , E. Shields, and M. Chassin. 1994. Improving the outcomes of coronary artery bypass surgery in New York State. *JAMA* 271 (10):761-6.

Hannan, E. L., A. L. Siu, D. Kumar, M. Racz, D. B. Pryor, and M. R. Chassin. 1997. Assessment of coronary artery bypass graft surgery performance in New York. Is there a bias against taking high-risk patients? *Med Care* 35 (1):49-56.

Health Resources and Services Administration. 2000. "The Hill-Burton Free Care Program." Online. Available at http://www.hrsa.gov/osp/dfcr/about/aboutdiv.htm [accessed July 25, 2002].

Hibbard, J. H., E. Peters, P. Slovic, M. L. Finucane, and M. Tusler. 2001. Making health care quality reports easier to use. *Jt Comm J Qual Improv* 27 (11):591-604.

Hibbard, J. H., P. Slovic, E. Peters, and M. L. Finucane. 2002. Strategies for reporting health plan performance information to consumers: evidence from controlled studies. *Health Serv Res* 37 (2):291-313.

Hibbard, J. H. 1998. Use of outcome data by purchasers and consumer: new strategies and new dilemmas. *Int J Qual Health Care* 10 (6):503-08.

Institute of Medicine. 2001. *Crossing the Quality Chasm: A New Health System for the 21st Century.* Washington DC: National Academy Press.

Kaye, N., and M. Bailit. 1999. *Innovations in Payment Strategies to Improve Plan Performance.* Portland, ME: National Academy for State Health Policy.

Kihega, A. (IHS). 15 May 2002. Personal communication to Barbara Smith.

Landro, L., Wall Street Journal Online. 2002. "FDA is urged to hasten efforts to require bar codes on drugs." Online. Available at www.online.wsj.com-Health.

MacTaggart, P. (CMS). 13 May 2002. Personal communication to Barbara Smith.

Markle Foundation. 2002. "News and Reference: Connecting for Health initiative." Online. Available at http://www.markle.org/news/_news_pressrelease_062102.stm [accessed Sept. 26, 2002].

Marshall, M., P. Shekelle, R. Brook, and S. Leatherman, Rand. 2000. "Dying to Know: Public Release of Information About Quality of Health Care." Online. Available at http://www.rand.org/publications/MR/MR1255/ [accessed May 15, 2002].

McGlynn, E., and J. Adams. 2001. Public release of information on quality. Pp. 183-202. In *Changing the U.S. Health Care System: Key Issues in Health Services Policy and Management.* 2nd edition. R. Andersen, T. Rice, and G. Kominksi, eds. Jossey-Bass, Inc.

McGlynn, E. A., and R. H. Brook. 2001. Keeping quality on the policy agenda. *Health Aff (Millwood)* 20 (3):82-90.

McGlynn, E. A., E. A. Kerr, and S. M. Asch. 1999. New approach to assessing clinical quality of care for women: the QA Tool system. *Womens Health Issues* 9 (4):184-92.

McIntyre, D., L. Rogers, and E. J. Heier. 2001. Overview, history and objectives of performance measurement. *Health Care Financ Rev* 22 (3):7-21.

National Committee for Quality Assurance. 2002. "NCQA Report Cards." Online. Available at http://hprc.ncqa.org/menu.asp [accessed May 6, 2002].

National Committee on Vital and Health Statistics. 2001. "Information for Health: A Strategy for Building the National Health Information Infrastructure." Online. Available at http://ncvhs.hhs.gov/nhiilayo.pdf [accessed May 14, 2002].

Office of Management and Budget. 2002. "E-Government Strategy: Implementing the President's Management Agenda for E-Government." Online. Available at http://www.whitehouse.gov/omb/inforeg/egovstrategy.pdf [accessed Aug. 15, 2002].

Paone, D. 2001. Quality methods and measures: MMIP technical assistance paper no. 9 for RWJF, National Chronic Care Consortium.

Pennsylvania Health Care Cost Containment Council. 2002. "PHC4 Homepage." Online. Available at http://www.phc4.org/ [accessed Oct. 18, 2002].

Rollman, B. L., B. H. Hanusa, T. Gilbert, H. J. Lowe, W. N. Kapoor, and H. C. Schulberg. 2001. The electronic medical record. A randomized trial of its impact on primary care physicians' initial management of major depression. *Arch Intern Med* 161 (2):189-97.

Rosenbaum, S., B. M. Smith, P. Shin, M Zakheim, K Shaw, C Sonosky, and L. Respasch. 1998. *Negotiating the New Health System: A Nationwide Study of Medicaid Manged Care Contracts, Vol 1.* Washington DC: Center for Health Policy Research, The George Washington University Medical Center.

Rundle, R. L. 2002. "The Wall Street Journal Online: More Health Care Providers Offer Patient Records Online." Online. Available at http://online.wsj.com [accessed July 12, 2002].

Safran, C. 2001. msJAMA. Electronic medical records: a decade of experience. *JAMA* 285 (13):1766.

Schauffler, H. H., and J. K. Mordavsky. 2001. Consumer reports in health care: do they make a difference. *Annu Rev Public Health* 22:69-89.

Schneider, E. C., and T. Lieberman. 2001. Publicly disclosed information about the quality of health care: response of the U.S. public. *Qual Health Care* 10 (2):96-103.

Schneider, E. C., V. Riehl, S. Courte-Wienecke, D. M. Eddy, and C. Sennett. 1999. Enhancing performance measurement: NCQA's road map for a health information framework. National Committee for Quality Assurance. *JAMA* 282 (12):1184-90.

Scientific Registry of Transplant Recipients. 2001. "ustransplant.org - Transplant Statistics - Annual Report." Online. Available at http://www.ustransplant.org/annual_reports/ar02/ar01_appendixh.html [accessed Sept. 30, 2002].

Simon, L. P., and A. F. Monroe. 2001. California provider group report cards: what do they tell us? *Am J Med Qual* 16 (2):61-70.

Webster, S. A. 2001. "Detroit News Online: Hospitals Slow to Adopt Electronic Drug System." Online. Available at www.detroitnews.com/2001/0107/09/a01-245238.htm [accessed July 3, 2002].

6

A Research Agenda to Support Quality Enhancement Processes

Summary of Chapter Recommendations

Implementation and evaluation of a national quality enhancement strategy focused on the use of standardized performance measures to monitor and improve quality will require a robust applied health services research capacity. Steps should be taken to ensure that the health services research agendas developed by the various government programs are complementary; address the salient concerns and needs of the populations served and of their care providers; and advance the capabilities of the government health programs in the roles of regulators, purchasers, and providers to promote excellence in health care.

Recommendation 8: The government health care programs should work together to develop a comprehensive health services research agenda that will support the quality enhancement processes of all programs. The Quality Interagency Coordination (QuIC) Task Force (or some similar interdepartmental structure with representation from each of the government health care programs and the Agency for Healthcare Research and Quality [AHRQ]) should be provided the authority and resources needed to carry out this responsibility. This agenda for fiscal years (FY) 2003–2005 should support the following:
   a. Establishment of core sets of standardized performance measures
   b. Ongoing evaluation of the impact of the use of standardized performance measurement and reporting by the six major government health care programs

c. Development and evaluation of specific strategies that can be used to improve the federal government's capability to leverage its purchaser, regulator, and provider roles to enhance quality
d. Monitoring of national progress in meeting the six national quality aims (safety, effectiveness, patient-centeredness, timeliness, efficiency, and equity)

The QuIC membership should ensure that the experience of the states and the needs of the populations served by Medicaid and SCHIP are reflected in the research agenda. AHRQ should continue to staff the QuIC and provide the organizational locus of QuIC research activity.

Additional public investments in independent health services research will be critical to both the development and the implementation of the research agenda by the AHRQ and the six major government health care programs. Congress should ensure that the institutional organization and appropriations for health services research are adequate to meet this important objective.

This chapter presents the committee's view of a research agenda to support the quality enhancement processes of the government health care programs. It begins with an overview of the current research activities supported by the federal government. The need for coordination of these activities is then discussed. The final section outlines what the committee believes to be the critical research priorities in health care quality.

OVERVIEW OF CURRENT RESEARCH ACTIVITIES

The federal government provides extensive support for four types of health research: laboratory research, clinical research, population-based epidemiological and environmental research, and applied health services research. Laboratory and clinical research is conducted mainly by the National Institutes of Health (NIH) (2002a), which operated in 2001 with a budget of approximately $20 billion. The Centers for Disease Control and Prevention (CDC) (2002), with a 2001 operating budget of approximately $5 billion, takes the lead role in applied epidemiological and environmental health research. The Agency for Healthcare Research and Quality (AHRQ) (2002a) provides the locus for applied health services research; its 2001 budget was approximately $270 million.

For the most part, the type of research most relevant to the development and implementation of effective quality enhancement strategies is applied health services research. Health services research "addresses issues of organization, delivery, financing, utilization, patient and provider behavior, quality, outcomes, effectiveness, and cost. It evaluates both clinical services and the system in which these services are provided" (Agency for Healthcare Research and Quality, 2002e, Para. 2). This chapter focuses particular attention on research regarding the development of standardized performance measures, the reporting of comparative quality data, and the provision of financial or other incentives to providers to improve quality.

While AHRQ is the primary engine for this type of research, the Centers for Medicare and Medicaid Services (CMS), the Veterans Health Administration (VHA), CDC, the Health Resources and Services Administration (HRSA), and NIH also engage in relevant applied health services research and demonstration activities. Rather than providing a chronicle of past research that has formed the basis for ongoing quality activities, this section highlights some of the salient research activities currently under way in these agencies. This is not intended to be an exhaustive review of every current quality-related project, but to provide a flavor of the range and types of initiatives being undertaken that are relevant to this report.

Agency for Healthcare Research and Quality

Created by statute in 1989 as the Agency for Health Care Policy and Research, AHRQ administers programs and activities across a range of policy concerns, from access, to care, to cost-effectiveness, to quality of care. Its activities are organized under six separate research centers: the Center for Cost and Financial Studies, Center for Organization and Delivery Studies, Center for Primary Care Research, Center for Practice and Technology Assessment, Center for Outcomes and Effectiveness, and Center for Quality Improvement and Patient Safety. Much of the work related to the development of performance measures and tools, a small part of AHRQ's overall mission, is conducted by the last center (Agency for Healthcare Research and Quality, 2001).

AHRQ funds both commissioned and investigator-initiated research efforts designed to enhance quality measurement and improve care. The quality-related research ranges from outcomes research, to performance measurement, to patient safety initiatives. For example, included in the safety agenda are 24 projects examining different methods of collecting and analyzing data to identify factors that create a higher risk of medical errors, 22 projects analyzing how computer technology can be used to reduce errors and improve the quality of care, 8 projects exploring the effects of working conditions on patient safety, and 23 projects focusing on the development of new strategies to improve patient safety at health care facilities (Agency for Healthcare Research and Quality, 2001).

In addition to its line of research on patient safety, AHRQ coordinates research initiatives directly related to performance measurement for quality improvement. These initiatives fall into three general categories: synthesizing the evidence to enable the development of guidelines and performance measures, enabling provider awareness of and response to clinical information, and improving the usefulness of comparative quality information made publicly available.

Evidence-based practice centers operating from 12 research and medical centers around the country (Agency for Healthcare Research and Quality, 2002c) synthesize and distill the clinical evidence on interventions for specified conditions. The objective is to provide organizations with a basis for the development of clinical guidelines and in some cases to enable the translation of the available clinical consensus into valid performance standards (Agency for Healthcare Research and Quality, 2002d). This translation process occurs through Q-Span, a project designed to expand the scope of valid, ready-to-use measures through cooperative research agreements.

Q-Span, due to be completed in FY 2003, develops and tests performance measures for specific conditions, patient populations, and care settings. Measures validated through the Q-Span project will be added to CONQUEST, an AHRQ compilation of over 1200 existing performance measures that can be searched by topic by providers, researchers, and patients (Agency for Healthcare Research and Quality, 2002b). The Q-Span project is intended to develop or modify measures for use in different settings and populations, thereby filling identified measurement gaps. Measures from the Q-Span project, CONQUEST, and other research will be incorporated into the National Measures Clearinghouse, previously developed through an AHRQ contract.

While not engaged specifically in the development of performance measures, AHRQ's Patient Outcomes Research Team (PORT) evaluates interventions for particular illnesses and conditions and formulates recommendations based on evidence from multiyear studies of which strategies achieve the best outcomes. For example, AHRQ has coordinated PORT studies on asthma, low birth weight, pneumonia, depression, schizophrenia, prostate disease, cataract surgery, dialysis care, and breast cancer (Agency for Healthcare Research and Quality, 1998).

The Translating Research Into Practice (TRIP) initiative focuses on developing strategies to shorten the time lag between publication of research findings and incorporation of those findings into routine clinical practice. The average amount of time required for research findings to affect direct patient care can be as long as two decades (Agency for Healthcare Research and Quality, 2000). TRIP's purpose, divided into two phases, is to evaluate research dissemination models and tools for their effectiveness in bringing about changes in practice. The 14 projects under TRIP I focus on strategies for collecting data, while the 27 projects under TRIP II examine implementation strategies and their effectiveness in achieving practice changes among providers with different characteristics and clinical populations across diverse settings (Agency for Healthcare Research and Quality, 2000).

In addition to performance and outcome measurement, there has recently been increased interest in improving the use of comparative quality data by patients, purchasers, providers, and policy makers as a quality improvement tool. As interest has grown in evaluating patient perceptions of the care they receive to inform the future selection of health plans, AHRQ has begun working to develop and validate surveys of patient perceptions and to display their results to consumers in useful ways. Research examining patient perceptions of care and its relationship to improved quality is evolutionary. AHRQ's development of instruments to measure consumer perceptions is an early step towards creating well-tested and validated instruments in the public domain to inform consumer choices.

AHRQ initially sponsored the Consumer Assessment of Health Plans Survey (CAHPS) to query Medicaid and commercial insurance beneficiaries on their experiences in managed care plans. As the role of managed care plans in Medicare grew, AHRQ and CMS worked collaboratively to ensure that the experience of Medicare beneficiaries would be captured in CAHPS. The CAHPS results are available on the Web and in print (Agency for Healthcare Research and Quality, 2000). The core of the CAHPS surveys is now applied to other federal programs and the private sector, with questions being added to tailor the survey to specific issues that may be more relevant to specific programs or populations.

CAHPS now includes surveys of Medicare beneficiaries who have disenrolled from Medicare+Choice plans to determine their reasons for doing so. A CAHPS survey first released in the fall of 2000 reported the experiences of Medicare beneficiaries in fee-for-service (FFS) Medicare. This survey was designed to enable comparisons of the performance of the FFS and managed care sectors as a whole on selected indicators within a geographic area. Through collaborations with other agencies and private organizations, CAHPS has also been adapted for applications by the Federal Employees Health Benefit Plan. CAHPS is the most widely used report of consumer ratings of health plans (Hibbard et al., 2002).

Research and development efforts for CAHPS are ongoing, and projects are currently under consideration for the second phase of the initiative (CAHPS II). Research is also underway to better understand how the information from consumer surveys can be used by QIOs to target quality improvement projects for providers (Garg et al., 2000). In the future, efforts need to be directed towards evaluating the usefulness of CAHPS and other types of comparative data and using those evaluations to improve both the substance and accessibility of the information presented.

In addition to examining and disclosing beneficiaries' perceptions of care, AHRQ has funded efforts to compile and make publicly available comparative data on clinical quality. For example, AHRQ has published studies on the comparative performance of health plans in cardiac bypass graft surgery, use of beta blockers after heart attacks, and asthma management (Agency for Healthcare Research and Quality, 1998).

Current efforts at AHRQ focus not only on improving the accessibility of publicly available information but also identifying elements of care that are significant to consumers and purchasers in decision-making. Because of evidence that the types of quality information currently available in the public domain are infrequently used by consumers and purchasers (Marshall et al., 2000), research is now focused on understanding the extent to which various stakeholders were aware of the publicly available quality information, and understood the information and found it relevant to the decisions they make. A great deal more research needs to be done in this area to support the efforts of the various government programs to provide useful information and reports to various stakeholders.

Responding to the interest in using financial and other incentives to improve care through performance measurement and public disclosure strategies, AHRQ participates in the Robert Wood Johnson Foundation's initiative, Rewarding Results: Aligning Incentives with High-Quality Health Care (National Institutes of Health, 2002b). Accordingly, AHRQ has issued a Request for Proposals to evaluate and analyze the impact of financial and nonfinancial incentives on improving the quality of care.

In response to a Congressional mandate, AHRQ is responsible for creating the National Quality Report, to be issued annually beginning in 2003. Developed in collaboration with the National Center for Health Statistics and other federal agencies, this report must identify areas in which health care is improving, declining, or remaining stable; provide evidence to identify care that requires more focused attention; and set forth national performance benchmarks. To develop the content and design of the report, AHRQ formed an interagency work group that includes representatives of CMS, NIH, CDC, the Office of the Assistant Secretary for Planning and Evaluation of the Department of Health and Human Services (DHHS), the National Cancer Institute, and the Substance Abuse and Mental Health Services Administration (Reilly, 2001). This collaboration reflects AHRQ's organizational and technical assistance experience in working with other agencies within DHHS.

Finally, AHRQ currently provides administrative support to the QuIC

Task Force. In addition to its coordination functions, described in Chapter 4, QuIC sponsors a number of research activities together with AHRQ and other agencies that are funded by the participating agencies. For example, QuIC works with AHRQ to develop risk adjustment methods for performance measurement and collaborates with the Department of Labor in exploring the effects of working conditions in health care institutions on patient safety (Agency for Healthcare Research and Quality, 2001; Eisenberg et al., 2001). By staffing QuIC in its implementation activities, AHRQ has expanded the contexts for collaboration with other agencies. These activities support the committee's recommended role for AHRQ in working with QuIC to coordinate research.

Centers for Medicare and Medicaid Services

Charged with administering Medicare, Medicaid, and the State Children's' Health Insurance Program (SCHIP), CMS focuses on the conduct of measurement and improvement activities. In addition to its implementation activities, however, CMS engages in a number of quality-related research initiatives, many of which are undertaken in collaboration with AHRQ. Because Medicare is the largest payer in the federal government, CMS has been able to use demonstration projects with providers to test quality improvement and performance models. Its research efforts generally fall into three categories, development and testing of: performance measures, outcomes measures, and more accessible, consumer-oriented comparative quality information on Medicare providers and contractors. Reflecting the increasing prevalence of chronic illness and its implications for future care needs (see Chapter 2), much of this research focuses on quality oversight in nonacute settings, such as nursing homes and home care. Research on nonacute settings presents an opportunity for evaluating the integration of quality oversight across setting and providers.

The Diabetes Quality Improvement Project (DQIP), sponsored by CMS, represents one of the largest demonstration projects on performance measurement. In a collaborative effort involving CMS, patient advocacy groups, private-sector quality organizations, providers, researchers, and other government agencies, DQIP identified seven core measures for diabetes care, streamlining the multiplicity of measures for diabetes (see Appendix B). It then created a toolbox to implement a measurement and reporting process. The DQIP performance measures have been adopted by the larger federal health programs and are implemented in all 50 states (Fleming et al., 2001). The Study of Clinically Relevant Indicators for Pharmacologic Therapy (SCRIPT) is using the same public–private collaboration model in a demonstration project to develop a core set of standardized performance measures for use in a variety of settings for medication management of atrial fibrillation, congestive heart failure, coronary artery disease, diabetes, dyslipidemia, hypertension, and post–myocardial infarction (Fleming, 2001).

As part of the QIO Seventh Scope of Work (see Chapter 4), CMS developed a home care demonstration project to test the Outcomes-Based Quality Improvement Technology, a systematic approach to measuring outcomes and targeting care processes that require improvement in home health agencies. This technology enables the QIOs to work with individual home health agencies to identify areas in which outcomes across the patient census are substandard, identify provider-specific causes of poor outcomes, and compare the practices of the home health agency with a clinical synthesis of best practices. Expanded to a pilot project in five states, the Outcomes-Based Quality Improvement Technology collaboration operates with a 67 percent participation rate by home health agencies (Thoumaian, 2002).

In addition to these major demonstration initiatives, the Health Care Quality Improvement Program, implemented by the QIOs, formulates evidence-based performance measures for use in its initiatives, primarily in Medicare, to improve care. The QIO Support Centers project engages in a synthesis of the clinical literature around targeted conditions as the foundation for developing quality indicators (Centers for Medicare and Medicaid Services, 2002).

Substantial attention has been directed toward enabling better public disclosure of quality information. CMS has worked collaboratively with AHRQ to develop Medicare applications of CAHPS and is continuing research on how to format the results more effectively for beneficiaries. Assessing how better to engage beneficiaries in the public disclosure elements of quality oversight provides a focus for Medicare CAHPS-related research. Accordingly, CMS has developed a research agenda aimed at exploring beneficiaries' readiness to use comparative information and at tailoring information to the decision-making processes actually employed by users (McPhillips, 2002).

CMS has devoted particular attention to developing tools for public disclosure of comparative quality data for nursing homes. It began a six-state demonstration project in January 2002 to collect and publish quality information on nursing homes in Colorado, Florida, Maryland, Ohio, Rhode Island, and Washington. The data are based on performance measures developed through public–private collaboration by CMS, the industry, consumer representatives, and the National Quality Forum. The data collected were published in April 2002. The pilot is testing alternative approaches for public disclosure of data to determine which approaches motivate consumers to use the information and reflect the priorities of beneficiaries and their families (Musgrave, 2001, 2002).

Finally, CMS is developing a solicitation for a demonstration project to test ways of financially rewarding physicians for improvement in outcomes and process measures. However, the creation of financial incentives to improve quality has not been the focus of research efforts (Klauser, 2002; Treiger, 2002).

Centers for Disease Control and Prevention

Consistent with its public health mission, CDC has developed many projects for tracking the care delivered to patients, particularly when patient safety issues are involved. For example, it has created a voluntary system for acute hospitals to report nosocomial infections to CDC. It has also developed performance measures related to health promotion and disease prevention issues and established a set of performance measures to define expectations. In addition, it has created a number of performance measure sets for preventive interventions and screenings, such as counseling for smoking cessation, pneumococcal immunization for seniors, and colorectal cancer screening. CDC is also examining structural measures for quality through its Translating Research into Action for Diabetes (TRIAD) program, which is investigating the association of eight structural factors with quality of care and patient outcomes (Institute of Medicine, 2001b).

Health Resources and Services Administration

HRSA conducts grant and contract funding programs to improve access to health care and serves as an indirect provider of care. It has built an expanding community-based network of primary and preventive health care services. The HRSA Strategic Plan identifies four long-range strategies that are linked to the agency's research activities: (1) to eliminate barriers to care, (2) to eliminate health disparities, (3) to ensure quality of care, and (4) to improve public health and health care systems.

Accordingly, much of HRSA's research activity pertains to improving the delivery of primary care for underserved individuals and families, analyzing different delivery mechanisms for care, and identifying strategies for improving access to targeted areas of care. The agency's quality-related research has involved both its grantees and its direct providers. Current HRSA-sponsored research includes a study of the disparities between what is known about caring for people infected with HIV and current clinical practices, projects that demonstrate the efficacy of interventions for high-risk populations, and studies of service provision to improve the quality of care. The range of these activities includes an assessment of emergency room services provided to young victims of violence and an evaluation of the effectiveness of a quality improvement initiative for improving HIV care.

As with other agencies, two themes emerge in HRSA's research: obtaining information on patient perceptions of care and developing performance models for the management of chronic illness. To these ends, HRSA has created a patient satisfaction survey for its direct providers of care that differs somewhat from the CAHPS survey used by Medicaid; consequently, most community health centers (for which Medicaid is a major payer) must administer multiple surveys. Through collaboration with grantees, HRSA has also developed and implemented evidence-based chronic care performance models for the management of diabetes, asthma, and depression. In addition, HRSA conducts evaluations of the efficacy of its patient safety protocols. Significantly, the agency's research agenda envisions greater collaboration on quality-related research with other agencies within the DHHS (Institute of Medicine, 2001b).

National Institutes of Health

While applied health services research has not been the focus of NIH activities, quality-related health services research is conducted within each of the Institutes. For example, research to develop performance measures for care of depression emanates from the National Institute of Mental Health, while research to develop performance measures for cancer care is supported by the National Cancer Institute (NCI), and for Alzheimer's Disease by the National Institute on Aging. Reflecting its scientific and medical research mission, NIH focuses much of its research on evaluating the relative effectiveness of different clinical interventions and delivery arrangements in producing desired outcomes; developing clinical data to lead to the development of treatment guidelines; and improving public access to medical and clinical information, such as the results of clinical trials. Similar to the TRIP initiative in AHRQ, research efforts also have focused on strategies to improve the assimilation of research findings into community practice.

NCI's initiative on quality-of-cancer care includes identifying a core set of outcome measures for use in quality-of-care studies and strengthening the methods and empirical foundations for quality-of-care assessment. An illustrative project is the Cancer Care Outcomes and Surveillance Consortium (CanCORS)—a 5-year, $34 million cooperative study to monitor and better understand variations in receipt of quality cancer care and process–outcome relationships among large cohorts of newly diagnosed lung and colorectal cancer patients. CanCORS findings will complement quality-of-care studies based on data from NCI's Surveillance, Epidemiology, and End Results (SEER) registry program. In addition, NCI conducts an initiative on improving quality-of-care research within the institute's clinical trials program, enhancing the quality of care by improving the quality of cancer communications, and increasing the extent to which available scientific evidence on quality measures and assessment informs federal decision making on cancer care. The vehicle for this initiative is the NCI-convened Quality of Cancer Care Committee, which currently supports three collaborative translation projects with HRSA, CDC, CMS, and the Department of Veterans Affairs, respectively.

In addition to research on developing outcome and process measures, NIH examines the relationship of performance measures and guidelines to outcomes across different settings of care, thereby testing the validity of quality measures. For example, the National Institute of Mental Health conducts research involving separate studies to determine how the implementation of treatment guidelines for depression and schizophrenia affects outcomes and processes of care. It also tests whether evidence-based protocols for improving the quality of care for depression are effective across multiple settings and delivery systems.

The National Heart, Lung, and Blood Institute evaluates strategies that can be used in clinical practice to improve the implementation of national, evidence-based clinical practice guidelines for the treatment of heart, lung, and blood diseases and related conditions. Focusing on the delivery of medical care, this research evaluates the factors that affect the adoption of a selected guideline in community practice. The research is designed to identify barriers to the implementation of guidelines and factors that can enhance adherence to guidelines.

The Diabetes Research and Training Centers of the National Institute of Diabetes and Digestive and Kidney Diseases focus on developing and implementing approaches to improving the acceptance of guidelines. The purpose of this translation effort is to develop and test evidence-based diabetes educational modules, targeted professional training, and active community outreach.

Veterans' Health Administration

VHA has engaged in a number of research initiatives consistent with its use of informatics in the implementation of quality improvement strategies. Its research is structured through a number of programs and centers, including the Patient Safety Centers of Inquiry and the Quality Enhancement Research Initiative.

The Patient Safety Centers of Inquiry were created to analyze the elements of and develop better tools for improved patient safety. Located in

California, Florida, Ohio, and Vermont, these centers explore the efficacy of different systemic approaches to improving safety in major incident areas, such as patient falls and anesthesia-related complications of surgery. For example, the VHA Midwest Patient Safety Center (known as the GAPS Center, for Getting at Patient Safety) conducts research on the development of strategies for training clinical and administrative staff to create a culture of safety. Accordingly, it is developing and testing a portable training kit that consists of simulations of adverse safety incidents, blueprints for safety meeting discussions and the development of safety minutes, blueprints for team cross-checking to minimize errors by identifying categories of collaboration, and guidelines for developing patient-directed infomercials that enable patients to cross-check readily identifiable elements of different interventions (e.g., correct surgery on correct body part, discharge instructions). The GAPS Center also examines human–computer interactions to evaluate the kinds of errors likely to arise with electronic order entry and to develop mechanisms for overcoming the patterns of potential error identified through the research (Render, 2002).

The Patient Safety Center of Inquiry at Palo Alto focuses on the development of systemic solutions to safety issues found in workforce training, organization, and workload. For example, the center examines data comparing incident responses in hospitals with those of naval aviators to identify baselines for achieving goals associated with changing safety cultures. The center also develops cognitive prompts to avoid perioperative events and examines fatigue effects on clinical performance (Gaba, 2002).

The Patient Safety Center of Inquiry in Vermont investigates the effectiveness of quality enhancement activities around organized themes of intervention, such as reductions in patient falls and adverse drug events. Illustrating an essential element of quality-related research, the center examines whether or not specific quality enhancement activities actually result in improved care and better outcomes for patients (Weeks, 2002). Relying on self-reporting by quality enhancement teams at identified facilities, the purpose of the research is to determine whether the effects of quality-related interventions are sustained over a period of months (Weeks, 2002; Weeks et al., 2001).

The Quality Enhancement Research Initiative implements evidence-based outcome measures and evaluates the impact of efforts to translate the evidence base into practice. To this end, it creates a systemic approach to developing the translation and measuring its impact. Researchers identify the gaps in knowledge that prevent better outcomes, the reasons certain measures are not used by clinicians, and the manner in which clinicians use different measures. All data are risk-adjusted to enable assessment of outcomes relative to projected outcomes based on risk factors that range from severity of disease to patient compliance. After identifying specific barriers to achieving improved outcomes, researchers develop and test strategies for systemic solutions to closing the gap between actual and desired outcomes. Such solutions may range from improving clinician training to changing technical order specifications. In 2001, the initiative focused on modifying clinical databases to measure outcomes directly, rather than relying on chart abstraction, to enable nationwide assessment of the impact of the translation process (Demakis, 2002; Demakis et al., 2000). This research is facilitated by VHA's system-wide electronic medical record (See Chapter 5).

COORDINATION OF RESEARCH ACTIVITIES

Research efforts in all the programs have focused on synthesizing the clinical evidence base and translating it into quality improvement strategies. Common research themes emerge among the programs: identification of priority areas, usually involving chronic illness or safety for quality improvement; synthesis of the evidence base around those areas; and development of performance measures from the evidence base.

While the research strategies of the various government programs are similar, the committee believes greater coordination would be beneficial in the development of the research agenda to better support the specific roles of government in quality enhancement processes. Some of the research efforts are duplicative or overlapping. For example, HRSA has established protocols for diabetes management and surveys of patient perceptions even though the DQIP protocols and CAHPS instruments are being used in many other government programs. Appropriate applications of the same instruments in HRSA could provide a richer database for assessing the validity of measures across populations.

Programs that conduct relatively less research would benefit from direct access to the research of other programs or agencies. Such a synergistic relationship cutting across all programs would also permit more testing of implementation approaches by providing a broader array of contexts for demonstration projects—for example, to determine how different payment methodologies could be used to improve quality (Anderson, 2002).

Without such coordination of research, the implementation of standardized tools across the government health programs will be much more difficult, since the tools used may not reflect the experience and responsibilities of the programs. In other words, research coordination is an essential precondition for coordination of implementation. Greater coordination also is needed to conduct more retrospective evaluations of the effects of different quality enhancement strategies across the government health care programs and identify the elements of success or failure, similar to the retrospective research done by VHA.

Greater coordination would enable the identification of opportunities to include standardized quality measures and data elements in the design of other applied health services research. For example, the CanCORS project demonstrates how standardized quality measures and data elements can be applied in controlled clinical trials. Because of the substantial resources available to NIH and the advantages of building on well-designed trials, the committee concludes that spending should be realigned to encourage NIH to identify fields of clinical research for which the inclusion of development and testing of quality indicators and performance measures would be appropriate. NIH should engage in coordination between its various institutes to shorten the time lag between the development of research findings and their implementation in practice through more effective evaluation and dissemination of its own research. Consistent with recommendation 8, presented at the beginning of this chapter, these research efforts should be coordinated through QuIC with the support of AHRQ to ensure congruence with the efforts of the government health care programs to strengthen and streamline their quality enhancement processes.

Broad recognition of the need for coordination is already reflected in the establishment of QuIC, formed expressly to coordinate quality improvement efforts among the different departmental health programs and improve the consistency of oversight (Eisenberg et al., 2001). As discussed above, QuIC works cooperatively with all departments sponsoring health quality research through focused work groups (Eisenberg et al., 2001). The development of a comprehensive research agenda responsive to the needs of all programs should be coordinated similarly through QuIC as a complement to its implementation functions.

Such coordination would facilitate an ongoing trend. Indeed, it is the need to maximize reliance on core competencies already demonstrated that drives the committee's recommendation for AHRQ's role in staffing and housing QuIC. AHRQ already provides administrative support to QuIC, and AHRQ's director serves as QuIC's operating chair. AHRQ's current mission and existing pattern of collaboration ensures that coordination will reside in the entity with the expertise, infrastructure, and operational focus needed to achieve a coherent research agenda useful to all programs. An evaluation should be conducted by QuIC every 3 years to assess the usefulness of the research and the application and effectiveness of the new tools developed through this collaborative process.

CRITICAL RESEARCH PRIORITIES

AHRQ is already engaged in areas of research that are critical to implementation of the quality enhancement strategy recommended in this report. For example, the current efforts to better understand the information needs of various stakeholders and to develop reporting formats that respond to these needs should be expanded in scope. There are also new areas of research that should be vigorously pursued and will require additional support. These include:

1. The development of core sets of standardized performance measures that address important health care needs and reflect efforts to overcome methodological or structural obstacles to quality oversight.

2. The development and evaluation of specific strategies that can improve the government's capability to leverage its purchaser, regulator, and provider roles to enhance quality.

3. The monitoring of national progress in meeting the six national quality aims (safety, effectiveness, patient-centeredness, timeliness, efficiency, and equity) (Institute of Medicine, 2001a).

A wealth of performance measures already exists. In some areas, the challenge is to identify the best measures to be used across all government health care programs. However, there are also gaps in the performance measurement toolbox in such areas as mental health and end-of-life care, areas in which some believe inadequate attention has been devoted to measurement development. Lastly, there are important methodological challenges to measurement that must be addressed. Following are a few research areas the committee believes merit attention:

- Technical, organizational, and legal challenges to the assessment of quality in clinically significant areas in which existing performance measures may lack broad acceptance or appropriate data sources, such as mental illness and addiction disorder treatments.
- Methodological and organizational challenges to performance measurement for small groups and physicians.
- Methodological and organizational challenges to measurement of performance across different settings, types of financing and delivery arrangements, and time, especially for chronic conditions and overall health status.
- Development and evaluation of the impact of alternative payment models and specific financial incentives on quality
- Development of mechanisms for useful public access to comparative quality information.

This list is by no means exhaustive but is illustrative of the many types of issues that require substantial applied health services research attention.

Establishing Core Sets of Standardized Performance Measures

As discussed in Chapter 4, development of a core set of performance measures to be used by the government programs based on the common needs of all or most of the populations served would improve the effectiveness of quality enhancement processes. The research agenda must provide for the identification of appropriate measures, elimination of the multiplicity of measures that may exist for a given condition or intervention, and assurance of the clinical validity and credibility of the measures used (Anderson, 2002).

While many performance measures exist covering a broad spectrum of conditions and circumstances, there are areas in which performance measures may be lacking despite the substantial burden of the health condition or the characteristics and size of the populations affected. Adoption of performance measures to evaluate care for mental health/addiction disorders appears to be limited despite the prevalence and burden of these conditions in the government health programs (Anderson, 2002; Meyer and Massagli, 2001). For example, no mental health/addiction disorders are included for focused quality review in Medicare's Health Care Quality Improvement Program (Davidson, 2001). Similarly, while there is a substantial encyclopedia of measures for pediatric care generally, the evidence suggests that measures are lacking for the particular screening and counseling needs of adolescents (Foundation for Accountability, 2002). Research should be directed at identifying the reasons for the apparent gaps in adoption of performance measures in these and other areas, and providing mechanisms for overcoming the barriers to acceptance, including demonstrating greater congruence in the relationship between the performance measured and improved outcomes (Anderson, 2002).

As part of the national quality enhancement strategy, effort should also be directed at assessing the impact of quality enhancement processes in general. It will be important to evaluate whether actual improvements in care are occurring in the clinical areas being monitored and whether the attention devoted to areas of performance measurement deflects attention from areas of care less susceptible to measurement, such as care coordination among providers and between providers and community services (Anderson, 2002). Lastly, as discussed in Chapter 4, performance measures must be updated periodically to reflect the current status of clinical knowledge and to remain responsive to the needs of the populations served.

Addressing Obstacles to More Effective Oversight

In addition to gaps in specific types of performance measures, re-search can address broader structural issues that impede quality measure-ment and enhancement. The committee concludes that the following is-sues require careful analysis.

Performance Measurement for Small Groups of Clinicians

While substantial numbers of performance measures exist, the major-ity of these apply to facilities or health plans. The Quality Improvement System for Managed Care in Medicare and Medicaid applies by definition only to managed care plans. Most of the efforts of QIOs are directed at hospitals, nursing homes, home health agencies, and managed care plans. The only comparative quality information currently available publicly is for health plans, hospitals, dialysis centers, and nursing homes. Yet, a large proportion of care, particularly in the management of chronic ill-ness, is delivered from the offices of small group practices or individual clinicians—settings for which very little quality measurement exists.

The obstacles to systemic performance measurement at the clinician level are substantial. The decentralization and variation among clinicians, combined with the absence of uniform computerized clinical data, render data collection a complex and burdensome task. In many private-practice settings, it is not even possible to identify patients readily by diagnosis, a necessary first step in the calculation of many performance measures. Lo-gistical problems are compounded by analytical issues, such as how to obtain adequate sample sizes in small-practice settings to derive reliable measurements of performance (Anderson, 2002). These obstacles, how-ever, need not be permanent barriers. Because existing performance mea-surement techniques preclude evaluation of such a large portion of health care, the need for enhanced research to close the gap is compelling. Ac-cordingly, a substantial effort must be made to identify the most feasible methods for collecting data from small clinical units and to address meth-odological issues. The committee believes that first steps in overcoming these obstacles could include broader use of patient registries and data systems that permit easy access to clinical and other patient information.

Measurement Across Settings, Delivery Systems, and Time:
Patient-Centered Care

Most available measures tend to capture responses to time-limited episodes of care (e.g., stroke, heart attacks) rather than the elements of ongoing management of chronic conditions (e.g., ongoing communication between members of the interdisciplinary team and the patient, patient education and guidance for self-management, discharge planning). These "snapshots" fail to reflect the care patients receive as they experience it—from physician's office to emergency room to hospital admission to nursing facility to home care. Moreover, the data requested for each phase of care may be redundant or may not reflect the total care process. Creation of a common dataset from the nursing home Minimum Data and the home health care Outcome and Assessment Information Set represents an important opportunity to reduce administrative burden while providing more coherent information on patient care. Once data have been collected, substantial methodological challenges remain, including how to analyze processes and outcomes according to the distribution of care among providers.

Accordingly, measures that can be applied in multiple settings and at the point of transition between settings must be developed. There are numerous options for the delivery of rehabilitative and long-term care services, including home health, short-term rehabilitation hospitals, and nursing homes. Patients with very similar health care needs may choose different settings. The use of common standardized performance measures across settings would be most helpful in determining which settings are most capable of providing adequate care, and the access to such comparative data would better inform patient decisions.

Alternative Payment Models

Although the preponderance of this report has focused on quality measurement as the stimulus for quality improvement, the committee recognizes that measurement in combination with other strategies has the potential to produce substantial change. The use of payment strategies to reward superior performance (as discussed briefly in Chapter 5, with regard to information technology) has attracted growing interest; some states, private-sector purchasers, and health plans are currently experimenting with these strategies (White, 2002). Seven states provide financial rewards to Medicaid managed care plans that meet administrative, access, or quality/clinical care standards; 26 states employ financial penalties for failure to meet performance standards (Kaye, 2001).[1]

As discussed in Chapter 3, the committee recommends that the federal government take greater advantage of its position as the largest pur-

---

[1]The states using payment rewards to meet performance standards are Iowa, Kentucky, Massachusetts, Minnesota, Rhode Island, Texas, and West Virginia.

chaser of health care services. The means of determining the impact of financial incentives and identifying the amount and structure of payment necessary to effect change remain largely unexplored at the national level, notwithstanding a body of experience at the state level that could inform such research (Kaye and Bailit, 1999). Research is needed to develop different models of compensation (including criteria for qualifying for higher payment) and to test the models to determine whether such strategies actually change performance and outcomes.

The Rewarding Results initiative announced by the Robert Wood Johnson Foundation and AHRQ in early 2002 serves as an example of research designed to explore strategies for creating incentives to improve quality. It provides grants and technical assistance to purchasers and health plans to develop incentive structures that "align incentives with high quality care" (National Health Care Purchasing Institute, 2002). As discussed above, QuIC, in collaboration with other agencies, can identify those programs best suited to such a demonstration that would yield important information for policy makers across the various programs. AHRQ should devote increased attention to the evaluation of alternative options for building incentives to improve quality into payment systems.

Access to Information for Informed Decision Making

Evaluation and testing play a particularly important role in determining the best strategies for providing public access to comparative quality information targeting information for different users to ensure the most beneficial impact. While there is substantial activity directed at exploring various approaches to public access, experience and reliable knowledge are limited. Accordingly, this remains a somewhat experimental area, one that will be susceptible to modification and innovation as understanding increases.

Existing evidence indicates that consumers generally rely on comparative quality data only to a limited extent and make choices that do not necessarily correspond to their stated preferences (Hibbard and Jewett, 1996; Hibbard et al., 2001). Studies show that this lack of reliance stems from a lack of understanding or distrust of performance ratings and their perceived lack of relevance or utility (Vaiana and McGlynn, 2002). This conclusion is confirmed by experience with disclosure of comparative quality data on hospitals and health plans (Jencks, 2000; Schneider and Epstein, 1996). In the latter two examples, publicly disclosed data showing variations in the quality of care and patient outcomes have had little impact on consumer choice or health plan contracting with hospitals (Jencks, 2000; Schneider and Lieberman, 2001).

Current research efforts focus on developing presentations of comparative quality information for public disclosure that are more accessible to the consumer, creating greater incentives for consumers to use and act on such information (McPhillips, 2002). Recent studies suggest that performance reports must make cognitive demands on the user that are consistent with "the basic processes by which people make decisions," an element largely lacking in current public reports (Vaiana and McGlynn, 2002, pp. 3-4). Substantial support should be provided for efforts to improve the congruency between public reporting of data and the needs of users, including research assessing the capabilities of consumers to use the information and adapt it appropriately.

The committee believes that more education on the variability in the quality and safety of care, combined with comparative data in more accessible formats, will likely trigger greater interest and ability on the part of consumers to use comparative information on quality when making decisions. Early exploratory efforts point in this direction. For example, since 1998, PacifiCare of California's Quality Index profile of physician organization performance has disclosed 58 measures of clinical quality, patient safety, service quality, and affordability to consumers, and PacifiCare enrollees have responded by increased selection of better performing providers (Ho, 2002).

There is evidence that the behavior of providers changes measurably when they are confronted with publicly disclosed comparative data, although the evidence on the effects of such changes is conflicting and the methods used in the different studies vary significantly. Some evidence from studies of the effects of comparative report cards on the quality of care in cardiac surgery in New York and Pennsylvania indicates that public disclosure of comparative risk-adjusted data may have contributed to improved outcomes for patients, including high-risk patients; this suggests that some providers actually changed clinical practices to improve care (Hannan et al., 1994, 1997; Marshall et al., 2000). Similar findings are reflected in a qualitative case study of four of the worst-performing hospitals in New York, indicating that report cards combined with regulatory intervention for conspicuous outliers led to specific clinical improvements in cardiac surgery care. These improvements included increasing the level of specialization of providers and caregivers, changing the physical organization of the facilities, and revising surgical privileges and scheduling (Chassin, 2002). Such a beneficial effect failed to occur in hospitals whose poor or mediocre performance did not qualify for outlier status. Chassin attributes the quality improvement effects to four factors that he characterizes as difficult to duplicate outside of New York: the integration of comparative quality reporting into the routine regulatory processes of a government agency, vigorous involvement of the professional leadership, a continuous commitment to scientific evaluation of the program, and the "active engagement" of the health department as a "primary force for improvement" in a strong regulatory environment (Chassin, 2002, p. 49).

With respect to changes in provider behavior that affect access to care, Hannan et al. (1997) found that sicker patients did not experience greater exclusion as a result of disclosure of comparative data in New York. These findings differ from the results of an analysis of the effects of disclosure in Pennsylvania, where referring cardiologists reported in surveys that "access to care has decreased for severely ill patients who need CABG [coronary artery bypass graft] surgery" (Schneider and Epstein, 1996). These studies did not track the effects of changed provider behavior on patients who did not receive surgical intervention.

In a detailed, controlled study of comparative cohorts of patients before and after the use of report cards based on nationwide sampling, Dranove et al. (2002) found increased exclusion of sicker patients whose conditions were likely to require surgery to achieve health improvement, better matching of patients with providers (consistent with the findings of Hannan et al.), increased surgery on healthier patients whose conditions would have been more responsive to non-surgical interventions, and poorer outcomes (greater morbidity and mortality) among sicker patients who did not receive surgery compared with similar patients in control groups who did receive surgery. None of the studies examined long-term effects on health status.

The variation in findings among these studies points to the need to test different approaches to report cards and to explore the effects of these approaches in causing a broader range of providers to improve care, minimize unintended/undesired consequences, and support the interest of the consumer in being able to identify and select the safest and most effective sources of care (Hannan et al., 1997). These findings also underscore the importance of developing appropriate means of risk adjusting in publicly disclosed outcome information and promoting provider confidence in the validity of the risk adjustment. Without such risk-adjustment, comparative information could result in misconceptions regarding quality of care as well as incentives for risk selection by providers (Anderson, 2002). Accordingly, research should focus on the development and dissemination of risk adjustment methodologies that accurately reflect patient condition as an essential element of improved access to information.

As discussed in Chapter 4, research should be directed towards ensuring that the measures employed reflect important aspects of quality. Public information should focus on elements of care that reflect consumer priorities, address consumer assumptions about quality, lend themselves to easy and correct interpretation for making choices, and represent timely disclosure (Schneider and Lieberman, 2001).

The committee believes that structuring information to correspond to the core sets of performance measures across the six quality aims should provide the paradigm for research on public disclosure.

The relationship of process measures to better care and outcomes should be a defining consideration in the selection of the measures to be disclosed, and that relationship must be apparent in both surveys and presentation. However, the committee believes that because consumers make choices at the micro level of care (e.g. choosing a clinician) identifying and implementing an information infrastructure that can be used to collect provider-specific information for consumers remains an essential precondition for meaningful public disclosure of quality performance.

In addition to research on how best to design comparative reports to meet the needs of various stakeholders, it will also be important for AHRQ to better understand the potential users and applications that can be supported by the shared data repository (discussed in Chapter 4). The data repository is intended to be a more flexible tool for gaining access to quality information. In addition to requesting specific tailored reports, users might also access the data base directly and generate their own reports. A good deal of research and evaluation will be necessary to determine how best to structure and organize the data in the repository and to identify ways of assisting different types of users in accessing and interpreting data.

REFERENCES

Agency for Healthcare Research and Quality. 1998. "Strategic Plan, November 1998: Center for Outcomes and Effectiveness Research: Mission Statement." Online. Available at http://www.ahrq.gov/about/coer/coerplan.htm [accessed July 12, 2002].

———. 2000. "Translating Research into Practice; From the pipeline of health services research-CAHPS. The Story of the Consumer assessment of health plans." Online. Available at http://www.ahrq.gov/research/cahptrip.htm [accessed May 21, 2001].

———. 2001. "Quality Interagency Coordination Task Force (QuIC) Fact Sheet, AHRQ publication No. 00-P027 ." Online. Available at http://www.ahcpr.gov/qual/quicfact.htm [accessed June 18, 2001].

———. 2002a. "AHRQ Fiscal Year 2002 Budget in Brief." Online. Available at http://www.ahcpr.gov/about/cj2002/budbrf02.htm [accessed Feb. 4, 2002a].

———. 2002b. "CONQUEST Fact Sheet." Online. Available at http://www.ahrq.gov/qual/conquest/conqfact.htm [accessed Feb. 14, 2002b].

———. 2002c. "Evidence-based Practice Centers." Online. Available at http://www.ahcpr.gov/clinic/epc/ [accessed Apr. 29, 2002c].

———. 2002d. "Health Care: Evidence-based Practice Subdirectory Page." Online. Available at http://www.ahrq.gov/clinic/epcix.htm [accessed Feb. 14, 2002d].

———. 2002e. "What Is AHRQ?" Online. Available at http://www.ahrq.gov/about/whatis.htm [accessed Sept. 23, 2002e].

Anderson, G. 2002. "Testimony Before the Subcommittee on Health of the House Committee on Ways and Means Hearing on Promoting Disease Management in Medicare." Online. Available at http://waysandmeans.house.gov/health/107cong/4-16-02/4-16ande. htm [accessed May 3, 2002].

Centers for Disease Control and Prevention. 2002. "CDC - Financial Management Office Budgetary Information." Online. Available at http://www.cdc.gov/fmo/ fmofybudget.htm [accessed Feb. 4, 2002].

Centers for Medicare and Medicaid Services. 2002. "Quality Improvement Organization Support Centers (QIOSCs)." Online. Available at http://cms.hhs.gov/qio/1a1-c.asp [accessed Oct. 2, 2002].

Chassin, M. 2002. Achieving and sustaining improved quality: lessons from New York state and cardiac surgery. *Health Aff (Millwood)* 21 (4):40-51.

Davidson, E. (CMS) (phone interview). 13 August 2001. Personal communication to Barbara Smith.

Demakis, J. (VHA) (phone interview). 11 February 2002. Personal communication to Barbara Smith.

Demakis, J. G., L. McQueen, K. W. Kizer, and J. R. Feussner. 2000. Quality Enhancement Research Initiative (QUERI): A collaboration between research and clinical practice. *Med Care* 38 (6 Suppl 1):I17-25.

Dranove, D., D. Kessler, M. McClellan, and M. Satterthwaite. 2002. *Is More Information Better? The effects of 'report cards' on health care providers (MBER Working Paper 8697).* Cambridge MA: National Bureau of Economic Research.

Eisenberg, J. M., N. E. Foster, G. Meyer, and H. Holland. 2001. Federal efforts to improve the quality of care: the QuIC. *JT Comm J Qual Improv* 27 (2):93-100.

Fleming, B. (CMS). 1 September 2001. Personal communication to Barbara Smith.

Fleming, B., S. Greenfield, M. Engelgau, and L. Pogach. 2001. The Diabetes Quality Improvement Project: moving science into health policy to gain an edge on the diabetes epidemic. *Diabetes Care* 24 (10):1815-20.

Foundation for Accountability. "The Child and Adolescent Health Measurement Initiative." Online. Available at www.facct.org.cahmiweb/tee/teenhome.htm [accessed Feb. 19, 2002].

Gaba, D. M. 11 April 2002. Personal communication to Barbara Smith.

Garg, P., J. Lee, R. Hays, K. Kahn, and P. Cleary. 2000. Strategic plan for quality improvement using Medicare CAHPS FFS information.

Hannan, E., H. Kilburn, M. Racz, E. Shields, and M. Chassin. 1994. Improving the outcomes of coronary artery bypass surgery in New York state. *JAMA* 271 (10):761-6.

Hannan, E. L., A. L. Siu, D. Kumar, M. Racz, D. B. Pryor, and M. R. Chassin. 1997. Assessment of coronary artery bypass graft surgery performance in New York. Is there a bias against taking high-risk patients? *Med Care* 35 (1):49-56.

Hibbard, J., N. Berkman, L. McCormack, and E. Jael. 2002. The impact of a CAHPS report on employee knowledge, beliefs, and decisions. *Med Care Res Rev* 59 (1):104-16.

Hibbard, J. H., and J. J. Jewett. 1996. What type of quality information do consumers want in a health care report card? *Med Care Res Rev* 53 (1):28-47.

Hibbard, J. H., P. Slovic, E. Peters, M. L. Finucane, and M. Tusler. 2001. Is the informed-choice policy approach appropriate for Medicare beneficiaries? *Health Aff (Millwood)* 20 (3):199-203.

Ho, S. (PacifiCare). 29 July 2002. Re: Chapters 4 and 5. Personal communication to Barbara Smith.

Institute of Medicine. 2001a. *Crossing the Quality Chasm: A New Health System for the 21st Century.* Washington DC: National Academy Press.

———. 2001b. *An Overview of Major Federal Health Care Quality Programs: Appendix B*. Washington DC: IOM.

Jencks, S. F. 2000. Clinical performance measurement—a hard sell. *JAMA* 283 (15):2015-6.

Kaye, N. 2001. *Medicaid Managed Care: A Guide for the States*. Portland, ME: National Academy for State Health Policy.

Kaye, N., and M. Bailit. 1999. *Innovations in Payment Strategies to Improve Plan Performance*. Portland, ME: National Academy for State Health Policy.

Klauser, S. (CMS) (phone interview). 5 February 2002. Personal communication to Barbara Smith.

Marshall, M. N., P. G. Shekelle, S. Leatherman, and R. H. Brook. 2000. The public release of performance data: what do we expect to gain? A review of the evidence. *JAMA* 283 (14):1866-74.

McPhillips, R. (CMA). February 2002. Personal communication to Barbara Smith.

Meyer, G. S., and M. P. Massagli. 2001. The forgotten component of the quality triad: can we still learn something from "structure"? *Jt Comm J Qual Improv* 27 (9):484-93.

Musgrave, D. 2001. *HHS to Provide Nursing Home Quality Information to Increase Safety and Quality in Nursing Homes: Presentation*. DHHS.

Musgrave, D. (CMS). 7 February 2002. Personal communication to Barbara Smith.

National Health Care Purchasing Institute. "Rewarding Results." Online. Available at http://www.nhcpi.net/rewardingresults/index.cfm [accessed Apr. 22, 2002].

National Institutes of Health. 2002a. "National Institutes of Health FY 2001 Investments." Online. Available at http://www.nih.gov/news/BudgetFY2002/FY2001investments.htm [accessed Feb. 4, 2002a].

———. 2002b. "NIH Guide: Evaluation of demonstrations: 'rewarding results'." Online. Available at http://grants.nih.gov/grants/guide/rfa-files/RFA-HS-02-006.html [accessed Apr. 17, 2002b].

Reilly, T. W. (AHRQ). 7 June 2001. National Healthcare Quality Report: Background. Attachment to Edinger, S. Personal communication to Barbara Smith.

Render, M. 2002. Personal communication to Barbara Smith.

Schneider, E. C., and A. M. Epstein. 1996. Influence of cardiac-surgery performance reports on referral practices and access to care. A survey of cardiovascular specialists. *N Engl J Med* 335 (4):251-6.

Schneider, E. C., and T. Lieberman. 2001. Publicly disclosed information about the quality of health care: response of the U.S. public. *Qual Health Care* 10 (2):96-103.

Thoumaian, A. (CMS). 6 February 2002. Personal communication to Barbara Smith.

Treiger, S. (CMS). 7 February 2002. Personal communication to Barbara Smith.

Vaiana, M. E., and E. A. McGlynn. 2002. What cognitive science tells us about the design of reports for consumers. *Med Care Res Rev* 59 (1):3-35.

Weeks, W. (VA). 29 April 2002. Personal communication to Barbara M. Smith.

Weeks, W., P. Mills, R. Dittus, D. Aron, and P. Batalden. 2001. Using an improvement model to reduce adverse drug events in VA facilities. *Jounal on Quality Improvement* 27 (5):243-54.

White, R. Jan. 14, 2002. A shift to quality by health plans. *Los Angeles Times*.

A

List of Acronyms, Abbreviations, and Web Addresses

AHA	American Hospital Association (www.hospitalconnect.com)
AHCCCS	Arizona Health Care Cost Containment System (www.ahcccs.state.az.us)
AHQA	American Health Quality Association (www.ahqa.org)
AHRQ	Agency for Healthcare Research and Quality (www.ahrq.gov)
ANSI	American National Standards Institute (www.ansi.org)
APC	ambulatory procedure codes
BBA	Balanced Budget Act
CAHPS	Consumer Assessment of Health Plans (www.ahrq.gov/qual/cahpsix.htm)
CanCORS	Cancer Care Outcomes and Surveillance Consortium
CDC	Centers for Disease Control and Prevention (www.cdc.gov)
CDR	computerized data repository
CHCS I	Composite Health Care System I
CHCS II	Composite Health Care System II
CMS	Centers for Medicare and Medicaid Services (www.cms.gov)
CMS	Centers of Excellence (cms.hhs.gov/healthplans/research/mpqsdem.asp)

CMS Compare Websites:

	Nursing Home Compare (www.medicare.gov/ NHCompare/home.asp)
	Medicare Health Plan Compare (www.medicare.gov/ mphCompare/home.asp)
	Dialysis Facility Compare (www.medicare.gov/ Dialysis/Home.asp)
CONQUEST	Computerized Needs-Oriented Quality Measurement Evaluation System
COP	condition of participation
CPM	clinical performance measure
CPR	computer-based patient record or computerized patient record
CPRS	computerized patient record system
CPT	common procedure terminology
DBSS	Defense Blood Standard System
DHHS	Department of Health and Human Services (www.hhs.gov)
DICOM	Digital Imaging and Communications in Medicine
DOD	Department of Defense (www.dod.gov)
DQIP	Diabetes Quality Improvement Project (www.dqip.org)
DRG	diagnosis related group
EQRO	External Quality Review Organizations
ESRD	end stage renal disease
FACCT	Foundation for Accountability (www.facct.org)
FDA	Food and Drug Administration (www.fda.gov)
FFS	fee-for-service
FFY	federal fiscal year
FHIE	Federal Health Information Exchange
FPL	federal poverty level
HCFA	Health Care Financing Agency (now called CMS, see above)
HEDIS	Health Plan Employer Data and Information Set (www.ncqa.org/programs/hedis/index.htm)
HIS	health information system
HIV/AIDS	human immunodeficiency virus/acquired immunodeficiency syndrome
HOS	Health Outcomes Survey

HRSA	Health Resources and Services Administration (www.hrsa.gov)
ICD	International Classification of Diseases
IHS	Indian Health Service (www.ihs.gov)
IOM	Institute of Medicine (www.iom.edu)
IT	information technology
JCAHO	Joint Commission on Accreditation of Healthcare Organizations (www.jcaho.org)
KePRO	Keystone Peer Review Organization (www.kepro.org)
LOINC	logical observation identifiers, names and codes
MDS	minimum data set
MedPAC	Medicare Payment Advisory Commission (www.medpac.gov)
MEPS	Medical Expenditure Panel Survey (www.meps.ahrq.gov)
MHS	Military Health System
MSIS	Medicaid Statistical Information Set
MTF	military treatment facility
MUMPS	Massachusetts General Hospital Utility Multi-Programming System
NCI	National Cancer Institute (www.nci.nih.gov)
NCPDP	National Council for Prescription Drug Programs (www.ncpdp.org)
NCPS	National Center for Patient Safety (www.patientsafety.gov)
NCQA	National Committee for Quality Assurance (www.ncqa.org)
NCVHS	National Committee on Vital and Health Statistics (www.ncvhs.hhs.gov)
NDC	National Drug Codes
NHCPI	National Health Care Purchasing Institute (www.nhcpi.net)
NIH	National Institutes of Health (www.nih.gov)
NQF	National Quality Forum (www.qualityforum.gov)
NSQIP	National Surgical Quality Improvement Program (www.nsqip.org)

OASIS	Outcome Assessment and Information Set
OPM	U.S. Office of Personnel Management (www.opm.gov)
ORYX	JCAHO's performance measurement initiative (www.jcaho.org/pms/index.htm)
PCC	patient care component
PHC4	Pennsylvania Health Care Cost Containment Council (www.phc4.org)
PORT	patient outcome research team
PSTF	Patient Safety Task Force
QA	quality assurance
QIO	Quality Improvement Organization
Q-Span	expansion of quality of care measures
QUERI	Quality Enhancement Research Initiative
QuIC	Quality Interagency Coordination Task Force (www.quic.gov)
QUISMC	Quality Improvement System for Managed Care
SCHIP	State Children's Health Insurance Program (www.cms.gov/schip/default.asp)
SCRIPT	Study of Clinically Relevant Indicators for Pharmacologic Therapy
SEER	Surveillance, Epidemiology, and End Results
SNOMED	Systemized Nomenclature of Human and Veterinary Medicine
SSI	Supplemental Security Income
STD	sexually transmitted disease
TMA	TRICARE Management Activity (www.tricare.osd.mil)
TMIP	Theater Medical Information Program
TOPS	TRICARE Operational Performance Statements
TRIAD	Translating Research into Action for Diabetes
TRIP	Translating Research Into Practice
UMLS	Unified Medical Language System
UPN	universal product number
VA	Veterans Administration (www.va.gov)
VHA	Veterans Health Administration (www.va.gov/health_benefits)
VISNs	Veterans Integrated Service Networks

VistA   Veterans Health Information Systems and Technology Architecture

XML   extensible mark-up language

B
Adult Diabetes Care: Performance Measurement Set for 18- to 75-Year-Olds

Aspect of Care	Quality Improvement Measures (per year)	External Accountability Measures (per year)
Hemoglobin (Hb) A1c Management	**All Patients:** % of patients receiving one or more HbA1c tests. Distribution of number of tests done (0, 1, 2, 3 or more). Distribution of most recent HbA1c value by range: 6.0 - 6.9% 7.0 - 7.9% 8.0 - 8.9% 9.0 - 9.9% 10.0% or greater undocumented **Per Patient:** Number of HbA1c tests;[a] trend of HbA1c values.	% of patients with one or more HbA1c tests. % of patients with most recent HbA1c level greater than 9.5%.
Lipid Management	**All Patients:** % of patients receiving at least one lipid profile (or all component tests). Distribution of number of profiles done (0, 1, 2, 3 or more). Distribution of most recent test values by range:	% of patients with at least one LDL-Cholesterol test. % of patients with most recent LDL less than 130 mg/dl.

Aspect of Care	Quality Improvement Measures (per year)	External Accountability Measures (per year)
	Total Cholesterol HDL Cholesterol 240 mg/dl or greater less than 35 mg/dl 200 - 239 mg/dl 35 - 45 mg/dl less than 200 mg/dl greater than 45 mg/dl undocumented undocumented *LDL Cholesterol Triglycerides* 160 mg/dl or greater 400 mg/dl or greater 130 - 159 mg/dl 200 - 399 mg/dl 100 - 129 mg/dl less than 200 mg/dl less than 100 mg/dl undocumented undocumented **Per Patient:** Number of lipid profiles;[a] trend of values for each test.	
Urine Protein Testing	**All Patients:** % of patients who received any test for micro-albuminuria. % of patients with no urinalysis *or* with negative or trace urine protein, who received a test for microalbumin. **Per Patient:** Any test for microalbuminuria; if no urinalysis *or* with negative or trace urine protein, a test for microalbumin.	% of patients with at least one test for microalbumin during the measurement year, or if two of the three criteria for low risk are met, during the prior year; or who had evidence of medical attention for existing nephropathy.
Eye Exam	**All Patients:** % of patients receiving a dilated retinal eye exam. % of patients receiving other eye exam (e.g., funduscopic photo with interpretation or other) by type of exam.	% of enrolled members who received a dilated eye exam or evaluation of retinal photographs by an optometrist or ophthalmologist during the reporting year, or during the prior year, if patient is at low

Aspect of Care	Quality Improvement Measures (per year)	External Accountability Measures (per year)
	Per Patient: Dilated retinal eye exam; other eye exam (e.g., funduscopic photo with interpretation or other) by type of exam.	risk of retinopathy.
Foot Exam	**All Patients:** % of eligible patients receiving at least one complete foot exam (visual inspection, sensory exam with monofilament, and pulse exam).	% of eligible patients receiving at least one foot exam, defined in any manner.
	Per Patient: At least one complete foot exam (visual inspection, sensory exam with monofilament, and pulse exam).	
Blood Pressure Management	**All Patients:** % of patients who received a blood pressure reading at each visit. Distribution of most recent blood pressure values by range:	% of patients with most recent blood pressure less than 140/90 mm Hg.
	Systolic (mm Hg): Diastolic (mm Hg): less than 130 less than 80 130 - 139 80 - 89 140 - 149 90 - 99 150 - 159 100 - 109 160 - 169 110 or greater 170 - 179 undocumented 180 or greater undocumented	
	Per Patient: % of visits that included a blood pressure reading; most recent systolic and diastolic blood pressure reading.	

Aspect of Care	Quality Improvement Measures (per year)	External Accountability Measures (per year)
Influenza Immunization	**All Patients:** % of patients who received an influenza immunization during the recommended calendar period. % of eligible patients who received an immunization or refused immunization during the calendar period. **Per Patient:** Immunization status.	None.
Office Visits	**All Patients:** % of patients with two or more visits. **Per Patient:** Two or more visits.[a]	None.

[a]This measure is not intended to imply an optimal number of tests or visits. Treatment must be based on individual patient needs and professional judgment.
SOURCE: National Diabetes Quality Improvement Alliance, 2002.

C

Technical Overview:
Health Information Systems of
VHA and DOD

Following is a brief technical description of the IT infrastructures of the Veterans Health Administration (VHA) and the Department of Defense (DOD) TRICARE programs. The VHA and DOD programs utilize modified off-the-shelf technology and specially designed middleware to integrate disparate and legacy systems, as well as a consumer-oriented, Internet-based e-health model to support their patient population's communication and information needs. The heart of these information systems is the computerized patient medical record that enables electronic documentation of health data, real-time access to important clinical information at the point of care (e.g., radiological images and laboratory test results), and linkages to facilitate administrative and financial processing. Other applications such as those for reporting adverse medical events are spearheading the use of health information systems to improve patient safety.

VETERANS HEALTH ADMINISTRATION

The VHA has one of the largest integrated health information systems (HIS) in the United States. At this time, the system serves 6 million enrollees/5 million annual users in the 22 designated regions. The VHA's HIS is rooted in the five primary elements of its composition:

• **Architecture** that supports information exchange across multiple clinical disciplines and lines of business.

• **Computerized patient medical record** for clinical documentation and information retrieval.

162

- **Performance measurement system** that provides tools for analysis and feedback to providers for quality improvement.
- **Patient safety reporting system** to document adverse events and near misses.
- **e-Health communications system** to provide veterans with online access to their medical record and other health information.

Architecture

In the early 1980s, the VHA began building its electronic architecture using the Massachusetts General Hospital Utility Multi-Programming system (MUMPS) (Veterans Health Administration, 2001a). By 1990, the VHA had upgraded the computer capacity at all its inpatient medical facilities with MUMPS. Throughout the mid 1990s, the VHA redesigned its operational structure to standardize quality, facilitate access to care, decentralize decision-making, improve information management, and optimize patient functional status. In 1996, the VHA introduced the Veterans Health Information Systems and Technology Architecture (VISTA)—its current architecture that provides significant enhancements to the original system in managing day-to-day operations (Veterans Health Administration, 2001a). One year later, the Computerized Patient Record System (CPRS) was introduced to provide clinical documentation capabilities and to function as the center of applications integration.

VISTA brings to the VHA's HIS a client-server architecture that connects workstations and personal computers with Windows-style applications, to a centralized database. This system is commensurate with the architecture and applications used in most offices or at home today. The VISTA architecture is a compilation of software applications specially developed by the VHA medical facility staff (e.g., vocabulary), commercial off-the-shelf applications (e.g., MS Office), applications acquired through sharing agreements (e.g., National Library of Medicine), and corporate information systems (e.g., Oracle database) (Veterans Health Administration, 2000-2001).

VISTA provides a complete structure for all administrative, financial, clinical, and infrastructure applications in VHA facilities. The administrative and financial applications programs support the operations and management of the medical centers. Specific features include:

- Billing—automated exchange of veteran information between benefits administration and the medical facility, automatic coding of DRGs for inpatient care and CPTs for outpatient care, determination of fee-for-service charges.
- Patient management—inquiries for eligibility data and income

verification, record tracking to maintain control of records and radiological images, missing patient registry, patient fund accounts for holding/managing money while in hospital.

• Administrative—accounting and receivables management, audit reports, transmission and purge, EEO complaint processing, employee time attendance, tracking of staff education and training; engineering, equipment and facilities management.

• Safety—employee accidents with blood-borne pathogens from needles and sharps and body fluid exposure with automatic transfer to national database if necessary, patient incident reports for submission to the National Quality Assurance Database at the VHA's National Center for Patient Safety.

The information is organized according to patient or department depending on the needs of the clinician or administrator. To facilitate retrieval of veteran information, VISTA includes a master patient index database with the appropriate authentication protocols to verify staff access and restrict unauthorized areas.

Computerized Patient Record System

The CPRS serves as a unifying platform for integrating all patient-oriented applications (administrative, clinical, etc.) across the network. The CPRS is a Windows-type desktop applications program that displays all relevant patient data to support clinical decision-making. The CPRS enables clinicians to enter, review, and continuously update all information related with any patient. Important data, such as a patient's active problems, allergies, current medications, recent laboratory results, radiological images, vital signs, hospitalization, and outpatient clinic history, are displayed immediately when a patient's name is selected to provide an accurate, real-time overview of the patient's current health status before any clinical interventions are requested or performed (Veterans Health Administration, 2001a).

After review of the patient's information, clinicians can place orders for various items—medications, special procedures and surgeries, nursing orders, diets, and laboratory tests, etc. directly from the CPRS. The CPRS also has a special feature that allows the clinical record to be accessed in the operating room, with automatic generation of the post-operative report (Veterans Health Administration, 2001a). To address concerns related to privacy and access to the patient's health information, the CPRS is constructed with a method for identifying who is authorized to perform various actions on clinical documents.

CPRS applications include:

- **Automated order entry** for consultations and procedures that lets clinicians know of a possible problem if executed, and tracking and reporting results
- **Clinical reminder system** that allows caregivers to track and improve preventive health care for patients and to ensure the initiation of timely clinical interventions
- **Remote data view** functions allows clinicians to view a patient's medical history from another VHA facility to ensure the clinician has access to all clinically relevant data from VHA facilities
- **Health summary reports** that display patient relevant data, vital signs and measurements, etc., in a comprehensive report form
- **Adverse drug reaction** tracking with supportive drug reference software and a link to the FDA to report data
- **Hepatitis C** extract for tracking

There are a number of other clinical applications, some of which connect and/or import information to the CPRS. For example:

- Scheduling component for treatments, procedures, and follow-up visits
- Comprehensive applications for the major diagnostic areas including laboratory systems (with a blood bank registry), and radiology application with digital medical images and recordings of all kinds (e.g., x-rays, cardiogram) that can be accessed at the point of care
- Pharmacy application based on bar coding for medication administration, inventory accountability, outpatient pharmacy management, and tracking controlled substances
- Documentation module for home-based primary care, mental health notes, and therapeutic care by allied health professionals, and management of nursing care
- Immunology case registry to support a local HIV/AIDS database and an oncology registry in order to meet CDC reporting requirements
- Dental records for entering treatment data, reports and scheduling

Patient Safety Reporting

The VHA patient safety system considers both adverse events and close calls (events that almost occurred). These incidents are reported, evaluated, and used as educational tools for improving patient safety. When an incident occurs, anyone working in the facility can report it to the facility's patient safety manager who completes an online form to report it to the VHA National Center for Patient Safety. Incidents are prioritized according to severity and probability to determine if a root-cause analysis is required. Staff performing a root-cause analysis consider potential issues including: human factors related to communications, training, fatigue and scheduling; environment and equipment; rules, policies and procedures; and barriers that can lead to adverse events or close calls (Eldridge, 2001). When individual incidents in four categories (adverse drug events, falls, missing patients, and parasuicides) do not meet the requirement for a root-cause analysis, they are aggregated for quarterly reviews.

My Healthy Vet

In addition to VISTA, the VHA has established the My Healthy Vet program that provides veterans an online connection to their medical record. The Healthy Vet program is based on the online e-health system designed and implemented by the DOD Military Health System (MHS). Participating veterans are able to obtain electronic copies of key portions of their electronic health records. This record is encrypted and stored in a secure and private environment called an eVAult. The eVAult information is presented in an easy-to-view table format with direct links to more detailed and explanatory information to help veterans: (1) understand what is in their record and what they can do to improve their health condition, (2) add structured medical information in a "self-entered" section, and (3) enable access to the Health Ed Library that includes 18 million pages of information about health conditions, medical procedures, medications, recent health news, and health tools (Veterans Health Administration, 2001b).

Within the architecture, information is exchanged throughout the system using the ANSI accredited HL7 messaging format standards, a standardized reference terminology developed in-house, and a network exchange module that allows physicians to access patient information from any VHA facility (Veterans Health Administration, 2000-2001).

MILITARY HEALTH SYSTEM

The main components of the military HIS consists of:

- **Architecture** grounded in a core clinical database that supports information exchange with multiple other data repositories
- **Computer-based Patient Record (CPR)** for clinical documentation
- **Theater Medical Information Program (TMIP)** for medical readiness of deployed combat forces
- **TRICARE Online e-Health System** provides patients with access to health information

Architecture

DOD began implementing standard health information systems in the early 1980s with the fielding of tri-service laboratory, radiology, pharmacy, patient appointing and scheduling, and cardiac assistance systems. Each system was tested and implemented at 15 to 20 sites and provided the framework for future health information systems programs. In the mid-1980s, DOD implemented the Automated Quality of Care Evaluation Support System, which provided standard capabilities supporting patient registration, appointing, scheduling, and administration, as well as clinical quality assurance. This system was enhanced over time to provide a broader array of patient administration abilities and was expanded to include biometric/workload information (Military Health System, 2002a)

By the late 1980s, DOD began development of a family of information solutions, called the Composite Health Care System I (CHCS I). CHCS I connects medical departments, hospital wards, outlying clinics, laboratories, and pharmacies by integrating patient registration, appointments and scheduling with laboratory, radiology, and pharmacy order entry and results reporting. CHCS I architecture provides the pharmacy with drug-drug interaction warnings, laboratory applications links with over 100 laboratory instruments, and electronic radiologic images to clinicians. Currently, CHCS I has the capacity to document over 50 million outpatient appointments and perform 70 million prescription transactions annually (Military Health System, 2002a).

Since its implementation, CHCS I has migrated to regionally centralized databases in areas of high patient concentration, enabling the highly mobile military patient population to access their medical records electronically at any site within the region. CHCS I applications are supported by the MHS Data Repository, a clinical data warehouse that aggregates data on health plan utilization, clinical encounters and cost of utilization over the past five years from all military medical facilities worldwide as well as contracted MHS network providers (Military Health System, 2002a).

A number of applications within the architecture support administrative and clinical operations. The Pharmacy Data Transaction Service creates a centralized data repository that records information about prescriptions filled for DOD beneficiaries at 340 MTF pharmacies worldwide, the over 40,000 pharmacies in the retail network, and the National Mail Order Pharmacy Program (Military Health System, 2002a). The pharmacy service provides real-time checking of a patient's current medication list and allergies to identify and avert errors. The Defense Blood Standard System is a computerized processing and tracking system for blood products and services. The Defense Medical Logistics Standard Support System provides effective management of the military's global health system and the needs of active duty operational missions. The Centralized Credentials Quality Assurance System supports the management of the professional credentials for medical personnel, disciplinary actions taken against personnel, and risk management case tracking throughout the MHS.

The MHS continues to build upon the enterprise architecture and is now beginning implementation of the next generation of technology. The Composite Health Care System II (CHCS II) is the military's clinical information system that will generate, maintain, and provide secure online access to a CPR and associated applications programs. CHCS II provides the structure for a lifetime medical record from the beginning to the end of military service. The testing phase of CHCS II was completed in July 2002 for which pilot studies utilizing the CPR were set up at four sites in selected medical departments—Naval Medical Center Portsmouth, VA (Family Practice and Pediatric Clinics); Langley Air Force Base, VA (Family Practice Clinic); Seymour Johnson Air Force Base, NC (Family Practice Clinic); and Fort Eustis, VA (Primary Care, General Surgery, Internal Medicine, and Troop Medical Clinics). Full deployment of CHCS II will be facility-wide and scheduled for phase in on a region-by-region basis over a three-year period beginning in fall 2002 (Military Health System, 2002c).

CHCS II has three fundamental elements: 1) a seamlessly integrated Windows-type user interface (screen) for documentation at the point of care as well as the display of data derived from multiple external sources (e.g., laboratory); 2) an enterprise-wide, industry standards-based Clinical Data Repository that will serve as a "clinical warehouse" for the information contained in the CPRs and applications connected to the CPR; and 3) a migration architecture that ensures the ability to easily integrate innovative technology programs to the system as they become available in the future. By the end of calendar year 2003, CHCS II is expected to cover 37 percent of MHS beneficiaries, by the end of 2004, 71 percent, and by the end of 2005, 100 percent (Military Health System, 2002a).

Patient Safety Application

Within the MHS, if an adverse event or medical error occurs, the event is reported immediately to the supervisors and administrators where an investigation is undertaken. The MHS Patient Safety Center handles the investigations and all other matters related to adverse events. Its Website averages 1000 user sessions per month, and a quarterly newsletter on patient safety is distributed to 1500 personnel (Military Health System, 2001).

The MHS patient safety system is modeled after the VHA, whereby root-cause-analysis is carried out and used for quality improvement in patient care. In addition to the reporting system, queries can be performed on information in the Clinical Data Repository in order to identify deviations from standard practices or anomalous events in the data.

Theater Medical Information Program

The TMIP supports the medical readiness of deployed combat forces around the world. TMIP plays a vital role in force health protection by providing critical data for the clinical care of battlefield casualties and management of military medical assets. The TMIP system functions on an independent temporary database system that is linked to the Clinical Data Repository. During a deployment, the relevant medical information from the CPRS (held in the repository) is accessed through the TMIP. All clinical documentation related to local treatment during deployment is held in the temporary database. Upon return of the force personnel, the new medical information is downloaded into CHCS II and the Clinical Data Repository (Military Health System, 2002d).

TRICARE ONLINE

TRICARE Online is the military's e-health communications system. It is an online system that provides information on health conditions and interactive health tools, disease management and treatment compliance recommendations, a directory of TRICARE medical facilities and providers, and a communications system for appointment scheduling. In the near future, the online system will have technology capabilities for telemedicine and other e-health initiatives. The system is currently in prototype testing at five medical centers with a roll out to all facilities scheduled for late 2002 (Military Health System, 2002b).

If desired, patients can create their own Personal Healthcare Homepage to store medical information and resources in a secure environment. The application allows patients to create a personal health journal, store favorite links to health or wellness sites, and access disease tracking and management tools.

The Website also contains structured provider/patient messaging allowing patients to receive appointment reminders, request routine health tests, and by fall 2002 to refill and renew prescriptions. The VHA is currently utilizing TRICARE Online as a model for the development of their e-health system.

REFERENCES

Eldridge, N. 2001. *Presentation to the National Committee on Vital and Health Statistics.* Washington DC: Department of Veterans Affairs National Center for Patient Safety.

Military Health System. 2001. *Patient Safety Program. Instruction Document.* Department of Defense.

———. 2002a. *Reference Paper from Office of Interagency Program Integration and External Liaison.* Department of Defense.

———. 2002b. "Tricare Online." Online. Available at https://www. tricareonline.com/ [accessed Sept. 23, 2002b].

———. 2002c. *Presentation: The Military Computer-based Patient Record (CHCSII).* Department of Defense.

———. 2002d. *Presentation: Theater Medical Information Program.* Department of Defense.

Veterans Health Administration. 2000-2001. *IT Architecture.*

———. 2001a. *Office of Information System Design and Development. VISTA Monograph.*

———. 2001b. *VISTA and Health eVet Vista.* Veterans Health Administration.

D

Selected Agency Websites

American Health Quality Association (a quality improvement organization)	www.aqhqa.org
American National Standards Institute	www.ansi.org
Diabetes Quality Improvement Project	www.dqip.org
Foundation for Accountability	www.facct.org
Institute of Medicine	www.iom.edu
Joint Commission on Accreditation of Healthcare Organizations	www.jcaho.org
Keystone Peer Review Organization	www.kepro.org
Medicare Payment Advisory Board	www.medpac.gov
National Cancer Institute	www.nci.nih.gov
National Center for Patient Safety	www.patientsafety.gov
National Committee for Quality Assurance	www.ncqa.org
National Committee on Vital and Health Statistics	www.ncvhs.hhs.gov
National Council for Prescription Drug Programs	ww.ncpdp.org
National Quality Forum	www.qualityforum.org

Index

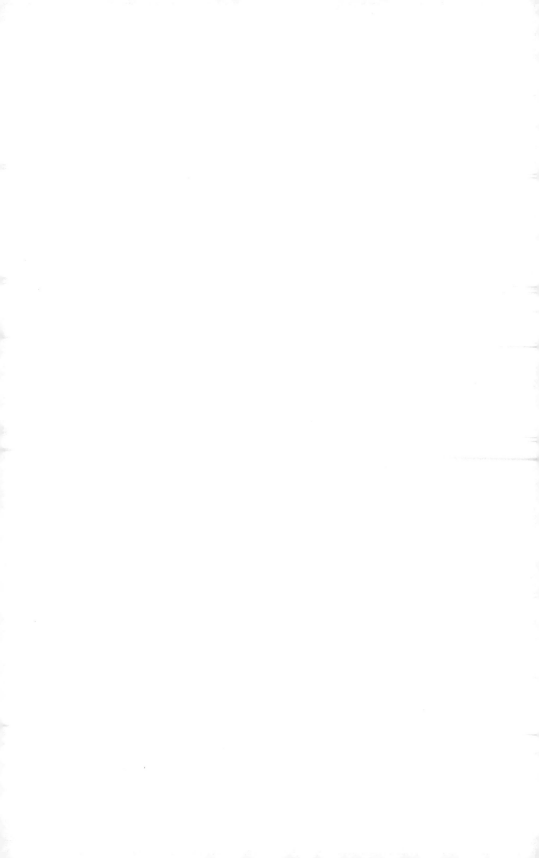